BEAUTY PRODUCTS CAN BE UGLY

The Hype, The Lies, The Dangers

ROBERT E ROCKWOOD

authorHOUSE®

AuthorHouse™
1663 Liberty Drive
Bloomington, IN 47403
www.authorhouse.com
Phone: 1 (800) 839-8640

Published by AuthorHouse 05/06/2016

ISBN: 978-1-5246-0644-2 (sc)
ISBN: 978-1-5246-0643-5 (e)

Library of Congress Control Number: 2016906930

Print information available on the last page.

Everything has beauty
But not everyone sees it

Confucius

Dedicated to my MOM
She gave me life
She gave me love to enjoy life
She gave me guidance to maximize life
She gave me the definition of the beauty of life

TABLE OF CONTENTS

CONCERN FOR MY FAMILY
GOT ME INTO THIS INDUSTRY

Being part of the beauty industry was the furthest thing from my mind when I started my career. I am a graduate mechanical engineer who started out working on Jet Engines for military aircraft and Fuel Cell Technology for the space program. Following that I spent the next 30 years developing chemical processing equipment and was fortunate enough to be granted over 300 international patent claims, more than any other engineer in the history of that technology. During those 30 years I traveled to over 40 countries on every continent working with chemical processing plants of all types to both teach and train their personnel on the most beneficial ways to not only install and operate equipment, but to increase the efficiency of their manufacturing overall. I put on seminars for hundreds of plants worldwide which included the attendance of thousands of employees from maintenance personnel to engineers to chemists to managers. It was during those 30 years that I was blessed to experience virtually every culture on this wonderful earth that we inhabit. I would be the first to tell you that those thousands of people I lectured for 30 years actually taught me more about life, the world and industry then could be imagined. I learned more than I taught. During those 30 years I worked with a number of companies that manufactured and formulated beauty products as well as companies that manufactured the ingredients used by the beauty companies. This was the time period that both enlightened and frightened me about the beauty care industry. I had the unique opportunity to go inside beauty manufacturing plants of all sizes and types. I talked to large numbers of product chemists and formulators. I talked to processing people around the globe. It was an education, few if any, will ever have. No University or study in Chemistry could ever teach as much as I learned during those 30 years. I learned what was going into the products and how they were being processed to become a final product that would be sold to you, the public. I learned what was driving the industry to go down certain paths. I saw toxins going into products; I saw processes that induced even more toxicity into the final product. It was not just in one plant, or one company, or one place, it was across the globe.

My family consists of a majority of women. My friends consist of a majority of women. As of now, women buy much more beauty products than men. With what I now knew about so many of those products I took my 30 years of training and started formulating products to protect my family and friends. I continued to study and increase my knowledge of what works and what doesn't. I also learned what was good and what was bad for the human body and being.

At first I was only making products, not to sell, but to be effective and protective for my family and friends. That philosophy eventually evolved into a company. I feel that in order to be completely honest and transparent with you, the reader, that I divulge that I am the founder and President of a company called Replenish Plus that sells 100% toxin free healthy skin care products. I am not the only company doing that but I take great pride in being one of the few leading companies providing those types of clean and green and effective products. At times I may make reference to some of my company products, but the purpose of this book is not to promote my company, but to inform you so that no matter what product you buy or use you will be able to choose a healthy, safe and effective product for you and those you love.

I felt it important that I write this book: not to frighten but to inform. To do the same I did for my family and friends. Knowledge is power, power protects. Hopefully this book will give you the direction and knowledge to protect yourself from the potential harm that can be inflicted on you by the misuse or misunderstanding of beauty products. Let us separate the myths from the facts; the truths from the misspoken; the harm from the good.

CHAPTER ONE
THE FINAL CHAPTER

I know it sounds a little strange calling the first chapter the "The Final Chapter." However, before you think I might suffer from dyslexia let me explain my reasons.

I remember when I was quite young (which was many, many years ago) and still in college, one of my school work assignments was to read the classic "War and Peace" by Leo Tolstoy which was 1225 pages long. That was followed by the requirement to read a second classic called "The Brothers Karamazov" by Fyodor Dostoevsky which was 786 pages long. Of course as we fast forward to more recent times, some people think today's classics should include "Harry Potter and the Goblet of Fire" which is 636 pages long.

As a result of embarking on reading such long books, I acquired the bad habit of compressing the time necessary to finish the book by either resorting to reading a short summary, which was usually written by someone other than the author, or in the alternative skipping to the final chapter without reading everything in between. At times I felt guilty for taking that action. However, I found I am not the only person who does that. In fact, there is a large subset of people who do that more often than not.

With that in mind I thought I would provide you with an author sponsored guilt free path to reading both the summary and the conclusions at the beginning. You could then spend the time that is convenient for you to continue reading in order to obtain all the informative details supporting those conclusions and offering you healthy paths to effective anti-ageing solutions. So let the conclusions begin.

Remember that looking younger can only come about if you look healthy. Any method you use to retain or regain your youthful looks has to be tempered with the primary need to not use anything that will diminish your healthy look.

The overall conclusion and truth that will be defined and refined throughout this book is the fact that 90% of skin care products consist of water as the number one volume content or ingredient, followed by a series of synthetic chemicals mostly derived from petroleum that make up the second largest volume of the product. It is usually way down on the list as far as volume content before there is anything truly healthy and straight from the plants or seeds of Mother Nature. The reason for this is unquestionably that most beauty care companies are extremely concerned about maximizing profits for their corporate shareholders and have an almost total disregard for the health of their end-user or customer base. Water and petroleum by-products are significantly cheaper to obtain than organically cultivating plants and then carefully extracting nutrient rich oils from those plants.

The beauty industry has been extremely successful at keeping government regulators at bay. Through a combination of excessive political donations and corporate lobbyists the beauty industry has kept government overseers and regulations virtually nonexistent. Here is an industry that is plying the body with thousands of chemicals and does not have to answer to anybody other than themselves as to the safety, quality, method of manufacturing or truth of claims made in their advertisements.

They can claim their products are anti-wrinkle, anti-oxidants, anti-ageing, or vitamin enhanced since none of these terms have any meaning or value.

Except for very minimal requirements they don't answer to the FDA, USDA, OSHA, EPA or any other government agency.

They can say things like "clinically proven" by simply testing one person in one location. There are no guidelines for "clinically proven". They can say "dermatologist tested" with their own staff dermatologist checking out the cream on a clam shell. There are no rigid "test" guidelines. They can say "doctor approved" or "doctor recommended" as long as they have one doctor on their staff or a friendly one they know. That "doctor" doesn't even have to be a medical doctor. He could be a "doctor of zoology" and be the one who recommends their products.

They can Trade Mark a catchy term like "Compound XtraXtra Young" for one of their ingredients, regardless of whether that ingredient is truly miraculous or just a different name for mineral oil. The Trade Marked name takes precedence and they don't even have to tell you what's really in that ingredient. Now they can make claims that they have a proprietary miracle ingredient that can take "up to" 20 years off of your age. The term "up to" is the legal saver. So what if it only makes you look only one day younger than you will look tomorrow? They have satisfied the term "up to". So, in your case, you are just short 19 years and 364 days of the 20-year miracle, but at least you are on the road of "up to" 20 years younger looking.

All of the above "tricks of the trade" is why most companies can and do use processed and/or synthetic chemicals to treat, reshape, change, color, protect and beautify the skin, hair, eyes and lips. In virtually all cases when a synthetic chemical is used to perform any function on the skin, the results are either nonexistent or short term effective at best. Please note that I did not use the words healing or healthy to describe any functionality for chemicals. Herein lies the problem. Synthetic chemicals may cover over a skin problem like paint covers over a damaged wall, but the problem still remains. Unfortunately, beauty products on the skin take it one more lethal step than paint on a wall. Many of the synthetic chemicals used not only don't resolve the problem but actually exacerbate the damage to higher levels and have side effects that create additional damaging elements with far more health threatening risks.

This is what the beauty industry wants to hide from you, this is what this book wants to reveal to you.

I will repeat the following throughout this book because I know that synthetic chemicals are never good for you.

SYNTHETICS ARE SINFUL

Our skin is our largest organ and either directly or indirectly connects with every other organ in the body. It has six major functions:

1- By serving as both a filtration system and a wall between our inner body parts and the atmosphere it protects our innards from attack by airborne bacteria, UV rays and many toxins that are in fluids which we either touch or immerse our bodies into.

2- Via its pores and ability to sweat, it regulates the body's temperature to keep it operating properly and serves as the exit door for accumulated toxins out of the body.

3- The nerve endings in the skin forewarn us of being in contact with potentially harmful heat, frigid temperatures or prickly incursions.

4- The thickness and elasticity of the skin serves as a cushion to lessen internal damage when we fall or are accidentally thrust into some external barrier.

5- It stores and distributes needed nutrients to every other organ in the body.

6- It is the only organ that constantly renews, repairs and rebuilds itself via skin cell generation and regeneration.

Refer to the chapter entitled **"Getting Under Your Skin"** for more detailed information and understanding of your skin especially as it relates to the ageing process.

Because it is the first defense, and in some cases the last defense, against both external and internal disruption, time can and will take its toll on the skin. We all start off with vibrant, healthy looking, wrinkle free skin. Every day when we look in the mirror, the first thing we see is the condition of our skin. When we see some of those perfections starting to develop imperfections over time we look for ways to regain that youthful, flawless appearance. For some it may be vanity, but for most it is the desire to look your best.

This is what the beauty industry feeds into. The ads, the hype and the claims make all kinds of promises and assurances that their method and product will make you look 10, 20 or 30 years younger.

One of the paths available is via medical or semi medical procedures. This would encompass injections and/or incisions as performed by licensed medical professionals such as cosmetic surgeons and dermatologists. This would include procedures involving Botox, Implants, plastic surgery and sculpturing. Other less intrusive procedures usually performed by licensed medical professionals and aestheticians includes skin peels, laser treatments and ultra sonic infusion.

It is not the purpose or within the scope of this book to discuss or analyze any of these medical or cosmetic procedures except for one caveat, if you choose to go this route, make sure you choose carefully and informatively. Make it your last choice, not your first.

However, the purpose of this book is to inform you about the pluses and minuses of after market beauty products that are applied topically to your skin.

There is no question that many more dollars are spent on beauty care products by women then by men. This is even truer in the United States then other parts of the world. Part of the reason is because of the fact that generally speaking, women tend to be more in tune with and critical of their looks thereby being more open to doing something about it.

It is probably genetic tuning over thousands of years that accounts for the differences between men and women, but as a man, and I may be wrong, but I believe there is a vast difference between men and women as to how they perceive themselves. I was raised by women, my mother and two older sisters. Most of my friends are women. I would be remiss if I did not denote one strong difference that I noted between the two sexes. There is no question in my mind that women are much more critical of their self appearance than men are.

When a woman looks at herself she is much more likely than a man to appropriate the use of giant magnifying mirrors and extremely bright lighting to enhance and ensure that she will see every flaw and blemish possible, even those not visible to the naked eye. Using these techniques even the most beautiful woman will find the most minuteness of imperfections.

Men on the other hand are happy looking into poorly lit fogged up non magnification mirrors after a shower or shave and therefore sees nothing but perfection. In fact, he normally sees Brad Pitt staring back at him.

Since the beauty industry is well aware of these differences between the sexes is the reason there are many more, in fact, infinitely more women's beauty products then there are men's beauty products. However, I will say that as of late some beauty manufacturers are more heavily pursuing the male market in the hopes of convincing the men that they also need some beauty care to look their best.

Independent of their market focus, every beauty company wants you to believe and therefore states that they and they alone have the miracle product to make your skin look and feel younger. In the United States there are well over a 100 companies manufacturing and selling skin care products into the multiple billions of dollars.

Regardless of all the claims made, in reality, other than medical and semi medical procedures mentioned previously, there are only three methods available to the cosmetics industry via topical ointments to make your skin looking younger.

1- Cover and Conceal
2- Plump and Plug
3- Renew and Repair

Cover and Conceal refers mainly to the family of cosmetics such as make up, mascara, eye shadow, lip stick, nail polish, hair dyes, etc... Unfortunately, many of these products do long term harm over time and actually may hasten the ageing process of the skin they are covering up. Please refer to the chapter entitled "**<u>Lips, Hair, Nails And Scent</u>**" for more information on this subject.

However, the main subject matter of this book is to discuss what is commonly referred to as beauty, skin care and skin repair products. This includes those creams and serums that are applied topically to the skin in order to effectuate moisturizing, anti ageing, anti wrinkling, anti oxidizing, skin rejuvenation and sun protection.

Approximately 90% of the industry uses method 2 described above as "Plump and Plug" to achieve their goals. In simple terms the creams and/or serums you buy have chemicals in them that expand under your skin to plump it up and are held in place by using another chemical to plug or seal your pores. The plumping expands and firms up your skin so that wrinkles seem to "disappear". The plugging is to hold those chemicals in place as long as possible, usually 8 to 10 hours maximum, before they evaporate or seep back out to the atmosphere. The reason for this being the method of choice used by most skin care manufacturers is for two major reasons:

1- It is the least expensive type of product to manufacture both from ingredient cost and processing cost, thereby offering high profits to the manufacturer. Based on my experience and knowledge, whether you pay $6/ounce or $160/ounce for your beauty care cream, in too many cases the bottle and packaging costs are more than all the ingredients combined.

2- It is the most expedient way to rid your skin of wrinkles and roughness. Unfortunately, the results may be quick but short lived; they only last as long as the sealant stays in place. However, the harmful side effects are not short lived. When you synthetically inflate your skin and seal your pores you disrupt needed natural body balancing functions not the least of which is your endocrine system.

The only way that makes sense to both diminish the outward signs of ageing and offer long term healing of both the skin and the body is to utilize the Renew and Repair system for your skin and body. It basically is a method where the body care product cream infuses your body with healthy nutrients which helps rebuild your cells to obtain revitalized skin. See the chapter entitled **"Plump & Plug vs Renew & Repair"** for full details and explanation.

Ok, now that we covered the summation, let's go into the meaty details.

CHAPTER TWO
THE SECRET TRUTHS

SYNTHETICS ARE SINFUL

The skin care industry is aware of a lot more than they want you, the public, to know. The reason for that is simple. The Industry has followed a tried and true paradigm that has been profitable for them and is the method by which they have set up their plants, their programs and their marketing. They may have learned a lot of new things along the way, but as I have understood, and the world has understood for many years – change is not only difficult but may upset the apple cart with which the industry and individual companies make a handsome profit. Most people who are in calm waters don't want to rock the boat of change.

The problem with that thought process is that like so many things, change based on knowledge is not only desirable, it is critical to the betterment of mankind, yet, in more cases than not, the changes don't come. I have always believed if you are doing the same thing three years in a row it is wrong. If after three years you have not learned how to do it better, you have decided to intentionally ignore your knowledge gain and continue to perform in an archaic manner.

Even worse than that is when you let cash profits become the focus of your being even if what you are doing is wrong instead of making cash profits the result of what you are doing right.

Most of the skin care industry does not want you to know the truths of what they know because if you did you would have the knowledge to be more discriminate in what you bought before you put it on your body and therefore would not buy the majority of the skin care products you presently buy. Alas, there goes the profits.

I will now list the truths and facts that the industry tries to keep under wraps. These truths will be expanded upon, dissected and resolved in the Chapters that follow. In fact, it is because of these

9

truths which I have learned over the last 30 years that induced me to write this book to inform you, the public, and to start a company that develops products to take all of these facts into account and correct them where needed.

Truth #1 – Water is the number one ingredient in upwards of 90% of skin care products. Water has virtually no beneficial effects except to reduce the cost of manufacturing and thereby improve the profitability of the product to the detriment of the end user. Water is the major cause of skin care product toxicity.

Truth #2 – 70% of sunscreens sold in the USA are toxic and can actually aid in inducing skin cancer.

Truth #3 - The terms "Organic", "Natural" or "Safe" means virtually nothing when used for skin care products and are usually misleading unless further defined.

Truth #4 - Generally speaking, the more expensive the product the more toxic the results.

Truth #5 – When the term "for external use only" is put on a skin care product information box it has nothing to do with reality. It is put there to protect the manufacturer not you the customer. If you put it on your skin "externally" it is going into your body "internally". The manufacturer knows it, the government knows it and you should know it.

Truth #6 – Most anti-wrinkle and anti-ageing creams achieve their results via a process known in the industry as "Plump and Plug". This process is extremely harmful to the skin as well as the body and eventually actually increases the wrinkling and ageing process.

Truth #7 - The detrimental effects of skin care products are much more harmful to women then they are to men. This is truly a major inequality issue for the 21st century.

Truth #8 - The majority of the vitamins and claims about those vitamins used in skin care products are false and in many cases are harmful rather than helpful.

Truth #9 - The most toxic ingredients in the skin care products are not listed anywhere on the box or in the company's product promotion. These are the hidden ingredients that a government loophole allows the manufacturer to keep secret from you.

Truth #10 - When a product has a list of so called "active" ingredients or "proprietary blends" it is usually used to mislead as opposed to inform.

Truth #11 - Cosmetic products and ingredients are not required to be approved by the FDA (Food and Drug Administration). There is no government overseeing of cosmetic formulations or ingredients or claims. In the USA only 11 chemicals are banned for use in skin care products. Over 1100 chemicals used in USA products have been investigated and banned in Europe and Canada.

Truth #12 - The ingredient list, by law, is supposed to be shown in descending order of volume content. The further down on the ingredient list: the less of that ingredient is in the lotion. There is one loop hole that allows manufacturers to get around that requirement.

Truth #13 - Many skin care companies still test their products on animals. This is certainly appalling to animal lovers. What is even more disturbing is why they use this method in the first place. It does not help humans.

Truth #14 - The most common preservatives to increase the shelf life of skin care products are the same preservatives that can decrease the life span of the end user.

Truth #15 – If a skin care product contains more than 10 ingredients, more than likely none of the ingredients are doing anything beneficial for the skin.

CHAPTER THREE
PROTECT THYSELF
NOBODY ELSE IS

SYNTHETICS ARE SINFUL

On average, a woman puts over 200 chemicals on her body every single day. When you add up the chemical ingredients in soap, hair shampoo, hair conditioners, lip stick, lip balms, shaving lotions, make up, rouge, mascara, eye makeup, skin creams, perfumes, and deodorants it is easy to exceed 200 chemicals. This does not include the additional 100 or so chemicals that are put on frequently but not daily such as those contained in hair dyes, sunscreens, perms, face peels, massage oils, bath oils and hair removal creams.

A man doesn't use as many so called personal or beauty care products as a woman, but still can easily reach 50 to 100 chemicals a day.

So who is checking out those chemicals to determine which ones are safe? Well, here's the scary answer – it's nobody that cares about you. There are as many as 85,000 industrial chemicals being manufactured and used by the personal care beauty industry. The first thing you have to know about the Beauty Care Industry is that there is no government organization that they have to report to before or after coming out with a product. Except in very rare cases the government does not get involved with beauty products sold to the public.

In the United States the FDA does no direct testing or confirmation of whether a chemical is safe to be put in a beauty product and applied topically to the skin. They rely on that determination to be made by the Chemical Ingredient Review (CIR) experts. The CIR is based in Washington, D.C. and was established in 1976 under the auspices and financing of the Personal Care Products Council (PCPC) which is the main trade association of the cosmetic industry. Aaahh yes, the fox is guarding the hen house.

The CIR, as well as the PCPC are non profit organizations and therefore do not file any forms which shows how much money is spent on testing. It could be a million, it could be a dollar. Nobody is saying or telling.

Let's look at one example of the CIR's overwhelming desire to ensure that every man and woman using skin care products are protected (In this context the word "protected" is not defined as "Let me cover your back" it is closer to "Let me take your shirt off your back"). In 2002 the CIR decided that it was safe to add phthalates to cosmetics. Basically phthalates are a plasticizer used to make plastics both more solid and more flexible at the same time. They are also a clinging agent. So when you put on creams, lipsticks, fragrances/perfumes, nail polish or hair sprays the phthalates glues the substance to your skin, hair and nails so that it will cling for a longer period of time.

Many organizations have determined that phthalates cause breast cancer, disrupt the endocrine system, and are harmful to the reproductive system in both males and females. More people in the USA are contaminated with phthalates then any other country in the world. The Environmental Working Group calls phthalates "cell killers". The Mayo Clinic suggests avoiding them. The European Union has already banned certain phthalates in nail polish and is talking about expanding that ban in many other cosmetics within the near future. In other words, phthalates are not good for you no matter what. In fact, because of their toxicity they have been banned in the USA for use in children's toys and child care articles.

The hypocrisy of that is the fact that phthalates can still be put in children's skin care products, including sunscreens. In other words, the Government doesn't want you to damage your child while he is playing with his toys in the house but it's ok to destroy his health while he is playing with them outside in the sun with his sunscreen on. Am I missing something here?

Phthalates is only one example of a lax attitude towards toxins in the USA. The European Union, which is not controlled by the chemical industry, as of 2014 has banned the use of over 1100 chemicals in cosmetic products sold anywhere in Europe. They still have a long way to go. But they certainly have gone much further than our FDA which in cooperation with the CIR has banned a paltry 11 chemicals out of 85,000. Although it is not the subject of this book, those same attitudes are allowing the use of many chemicals in USA food supplies that are outright banned in other parts of the world.

Even if you don't read another page in this book, that alone should get you very concerned as to what you are putting on your body and in your body. Knowledge is tantamount to protecting yourself because nobody else is.

In the cosmetic industry, as long as a product has a statement somewhere in their advertising that says "For External Use Only" or that "none of the statements made about this product is FDA approved" or this product is "not a medicine but only a supplement" they are government free and legally free to say whatever else they want to say.

Beauty care companies usually engage a slew of legal experts and/ or lawyers to make sure what they say can insinuate whatever they want to tout as a marketing claim but to put in small letters whatever they need to say to stay free of government oversight.

Look at the products you are using. Have you used a cream that states "It is for external use only"? That unto itself is impossible. If it goes on your skin, you can be assured that some of it, if not all of it is going into your body. Your skin will absorb it. In fact, that is the whole philosophy behind transdermal medication patches. A simple rule to live by is "If you can't put it in your body then don't put it on your body."

How many times have you picked up a supplement that promises all sorts of resolution and solution to various body or skin problems in huge bold letters and advertising? They then have a legally defined disclaimer in very fine print on the bottom of the box that says "These statements have not been evaluated by the Food and Drug Administration. This product is not intended to diagnose, treat, cure, or prevent any disease."

Really??? If you have no proof that it works or no intention to make it work, then why would you spend millions of dollars in advertising costs telling people how it does work? Is there a little hypocrisy here? Maybe there is too much hype and too little substance.

One sector of the industry that I find really plays this game to the hilt is the acne supplemental industry. Children, along with young adults find acne a major embarrassment and are willing to try anything and pay anything to get rid of it. The hype and promises are overwhelming, yet in most cases are underwhelming in their results. This doesn't even take into account the side effects of so many of these acne supplements.

For years there have been attempts at passing a so called Safe Chemical Act through the US Congress, but as of the time this book was written no such act has been passed. It is the author's guess that even if such an act was passed it would be so watered down to the point it would be essentially useless. A fairly decent Safe Chemical Act was passed in the European Union in 2007, but not so here in the USA. Environmentalists have been trying for years. Unfortunately, much of their efforts have been successfully thwarted by the American Chemical Council (ACC), a powerful lobbying group which is made up of most of the major chemical manufacturers.

When it comes to pesticides and pharmaceutical chemicals they have to be tested before they are allowed to be sold in the public marketplace. Of course even this system is riddled with holes that are potentially harmful to the end-user. The FDA (Food and Drug Administration) or the EPA (Environmental Protection Agency) does very little, if any testing of pesticides or pharmaceuticals on their own. The testing is usually done by the company that developed the product and wants to bring it to market. It is a little bit like having the criminal autopsy performed by the murderer. But at least there is liability if the product was declared safe by the company and then shown that it was not safe. The company knows they would open themselves up to both government and public lawsuits if they misled or outright lied about their product.

Unfortunately, when it comes to industrial chemicals, like those used in the beauty industry, everything is turned upside down. The chemical companies are very rarely, if ever, required to provide any government agency any information at all to assess the safety of their products. In the United States a chemical is considered safe until proven unsafe. If it is proven unsafe by a third party it can take years, if ever, to get through all the government bureaucracy and chemical company's resistance to making the changes to the laws that would restrict its use.

It is not the intent of this book to be a chemical course listing all the "bad" chemicals and where they are used. However, it is the intent to give the reader some guidelines and information about the more harmful ingredients used in beauty products and where to search for information about other ingredients used in those products. We will try to address as many of these areas as possible throughout this book so you will know what to look for BEFORE you buy the product. Generally speaking, one should always look at the ingredient list. If there are ingredients with names you never heard of or are too long to pronounce – be wary.

CHAPTER FOUR
THE LIES AND WHY'S

SYNTHETICS ARE SINFUL

Maybe I should have anticipated a little of what I was about to learn during my 30 years of working with the beauty industry, but then again, at the beginning I knew so little about the beauty industry that I never connected any of the dots until I had traveled down the road for a while.

Harry Houdini was arguably the greatest illusionist in history. He is quoted as saying that regardless of the true facts, "What the eyes see and the ears hear, the mind believes". Combine that with misdirection and you created an illusion.

In the musical Chicago there is a song entitled "Razzle Dazzle". One of its verses says the following:
Give 'em the old razzle dazzle
Razzle Dazzle 'em
Give 'em an act with lots of flash in it
And the reaction will be passionate
Give 'em the old hocus pocus
Bead and feather 'em
How can they see with sequins in their eyes?

Put Harry Houdini and Chicago together and you will understand what the Beauty Industry in far too many cases perpetrates upon its customers. To better understand today's dangerous direction of the beauty industry, let's look at the history of the tobacco industry which trail blazed the method of misdirection for industry and is followed by the beauty industry as it stands today. We will connect the two industries in a moment.

Prior to 1996 there was no regulation of any type on the tobacco industry, much like the Beauty Industry of today. Certainly it was not regulated by the FDA or any other government agency of any consequence.

Although Native Americans didn't smoke tobacco on a daily basis they did smoke pipes for religious and medical purposes long before the "white man" came to America. That may have been one of the determining factors that made tobacco the first "cash" crop grown in North America by the settlers of the first American colony in Jamestown, Virginia in 1612.

Smoking was common but not overwhelmingly popular because pipes were hard to keep going and rolling cigarettes was time consuming if not difficult. It was virtually a 100% male habit and looked down upon when women smoked.

In 1881 James Bonsack invented the cigarette making machine and cigarette smoking became chic and widespread. Several tobacco companies began manufacturing with the American Tobacco Company and Phillip Morris becoming the biggest by the turn of the 20th century. It remained a mainly male habit. However during World War I millions of cigarettes were given away free to American soldiers and since woman now were doing more work outside the home and making their own money the tobacco companies started marketing to the female population. World War II offered the tobacco companies even more opportunity to market their products to women. So many men left to go overseas that huge numbers of previously "men only" jobs were left vacant and had to be filled by women. Women become very independent, free of their husbands. The tobacco companies saw this as a great opportunity to promote smoking to women. It worked! By 1944 cigarette companies were manufacturing and distributing over 300 billion cigarettes annually. The government was allowing millions of free cigarettes to be included in soldiers "C" rations basically condoning their use.

The cigarette companies knew tobacco was unhealthy but that did not stop them from promoting cigarettes as being good for you. In fact, during the 1940's virtually all of the major companies put out advertising showing top name Hollywood stars enjoying a cigarette and telling the public that they should do the same. One of those stars,

Ronald Reagan would eventually become President of the United States. After all, cigarette smoking was "good" for you wasn't it, or was it?

The Tobacco companies were wealthy and had the money to sponsor the most popular radio programs and even invested into movie productions. Virtually every movie made showed the stars smoking. Advertising promoted the hype that even doctors recommended smoking. Lucky Strike cigarettes were being advertised as being toasted and therefore less irritating to the throat. In the 1940's they produced magazine ads showing that over 20,679 physicians highly recommended smoking Lucky Strikes.

Is this starting to look familiar? Doctor recommended. Good for you. Healthy for you. A wonderful gift for friends and family.

The tobacco companies of the 20th century, like the cosmetic companies of the 21st century had no government regulations or requirements to worry about. They could say whatever they wanted and do whatever they needed to do to make the sales. As was finally proven in lawsuits, not initiated by the government but by public class suits from the millions who were harmed and even killed by cigarettes, the tobacco companies knew what they were selling you was not good for you – in fact they knew it was outright deadly. Doctor's and public celebrities had marched right in tune with the tobacco companies, either because they honestly did not know better and were willing to promote even with a lack of knowledge, or they did know better but were paid handsomely for their positive testimonials. It took years of litigation and millions of dollars, but the truth finally came out.

I feel history is repeating itself all over again with the beauty industry. Lots of false promises, lots of hype, lots of doctor recommendations and lots of famous people advocating products that could harm lots of innocent people. That may not always be true, but it is true in more cases than it should be. With a total lack of oversight from any government agency or publicly recognized third party, the beauty industry can say whatever they want with little or no reprimand.

There were many times that I talked to chemists who were formulating new products for either their direct employers or companies that had contracted them as independents to develop the next generation of skin care creams and serums. After seeing chemicals going into the products that I knew were not good for anyone I would ask them why they were including ingredients that they knew were an irritant at best and a toxic at worst.

The response was almost universally the same – this was the way to get the fastest results with the highest profits and that's what they were paid to do and told to do. To get results it is quicker and cheaper to use harsh chemicals that peel the skin rather than using soothing nutrients that heal the skin. It is cheaper and easier to use a chemical to cover and smear the skin as opposed to using healthy organic ingredients that infuse and repair the skin.

What was fascinating to me is how many of them knew which was the healthiest and best direction to go but corporate bureaucracy would not let them go there. Many of them told me the right way to do things and I thank them for that. Those directions and inputs over 30 years showed me exactly the right path to research out when I started to put together my products.

People want to look their best and that is a good thing. What is not good is when marketers hone in on those strong desires and needs with a product that they know is not good for you but is good for their bottom line.

Not too long ago a friend of mine introduced me to a top social media marketing experts to potentially help me with promoting my product on line. This expert was affiliated with an organization that consisted of a number of social media marketers from around the country. I started to tell him about the health benefits and skin rejuvenation capabilities of my product line. Before I got two minutes of information out he cut me off. Basically what he told me is when you are promoting a product on the social media, the product itself and what it actually does or does not do is secondary. What is primary is you tell people what they want to hear. For example, as men age they care about their sexual prowess. Offer them anything that gives them the belief they can return to the levels they were at in their twenties and they will buy it. Whether it works or not is secondary. Make your money on the first blast and then next week you can promote another product under a different name and do a second blast. With women, they care about their signs of ageing. Promise them a solution, make it look credible and you got a sale. He told me if it doesn't work wait a few months and come out with another product and redo the cycle all over again.

I was aghast, not only was it totally sexist, but it was totally unethical. Needless to say I walked away. But it just reconfirmed what is done way too many times; lots of empty promises with few results. The real problem is not the lack of results but the abundance of side effects.

Let us educate ourselves via the following chapters so we can avoid not only buying things that don't work, but be aware of the side effects even with those products that do work.

The beauty care market represents well over $200 Billion in annual sales worldwide with skin care products being number one and hair care products being number two. This does not include the $11 billion spent in just North America for cosmetic procedures on top of that. Unfortunately, too many times the industry's drive to make profits overshadows the desire to make products that provide true beauty in a healthy way.

The reason I started this chapter by talking about the tobacco industry is because what they did was either intentionally or subconsciously used as a guide for many in the beauty industry. As was shown in so many lawsuits against the tobacco industry, they let profits get in the way of doing the right thing. Putting in more nicotine got people more hooked. Unfortunately, the more you smoked the more tar entered your lungs and we all know the side effects of that.

In the beauty industry, putting in more chemicals to get short term reduction of wrinkles and other signs of ageing gets people hooked. However, like nicotine, the side effects of these chemicals to the body can be even more devastating than the side effects of smoking tobacco.

The most common cancer for both sexes is skin cancer and the most common cancer for women is breast cancer. There is a rise in other diseases that affect our endocrine systems and the reproductive systems in women. I believe that part of the reason for this is because of the long term application of toxins we put on our body via the use of the wrong skin care products.

Let us stop that now.

CHAPTER FIVE
GETTING UNDER YOUR SKIN

Before you can do anything to help the skin, you have to know some basics about the skin.

Your skin is your largest organ. It comprises about 16% of your total body weight.

It is an amazing organ that is continuously at work protecting your body from invasion of airborne or liquid toxins, regulating your body temperature via your pores, cleaning out toxins via sweat emissions, renewing itself continuously through new cell generation, absorbing the harmful effects from an outside impact to all organs through the strength of collagen fibers and staying resilient because of its elastin fibers. The skin is connected so integrally to every other organ and parts of the body that many doctors can tell the status of your health just by the vibrancy of your skin.

Many people refer to skin as having only two segments, the epidermis and the dermis. In reality there is a third segment called the hypodermis. All of these segments have various layers within each segment.

In simple terms the epidermis is the outer protective segment, the dermis is the support segment underneath the epidermis and the hypodermis is the fat segment below the dermis. The skin varies in different thicknesses over various parts of the body. Generally speaking, the skin is thinnest around the eyes and lips, while being the thickest at the palms of your hands and heels of the feet.

Your total body is made up of approximately ten trillion cells. The skin represents about 1.6 trillion cells. The epidermis is like the sacrificial lamb of the body. The top layer of the epidermis, known as the stratum corneum, is made up of mostly dead cells to protect the living cells beneath them. These dead cells, which are mostly made up of a protein called keratin, which are the same dead cells which make up your hair fiber and nails, are being pushed off of the body at a rate of 30 to 50,000 cells per minute by newly generated basal cells which are constantly being produced in the second layer of the epidermis. That means your body is shedding about 75 million cells a day. Dust in the home consists mainly of these dead cells. The top outer layer of the epidermis is renewed about once a month with totally new cells.

As we age our body does not produce as many new basal cells as it did when we were younger. Also the basal cells we do produce are not as small and tightly formed as when we were younger. As a result, our skin starts showing signs of thinning out and in the worse cases are not as protective against invading bacteria which opens the elderly up to the potential of more infections. This can be minimized and/or staved off with proper nutrition both on the skin and in the body.

The epidermis is the thinnest layer of your skin and approximately equal to the thickness of a sheet of paper. In order for it to look wrinkle free and smooth it relies on the dermis segment underneath it.

As you can see from the skin cross section above, the dermis contains hair follicles, nerve fibers for the sense of touch, blood and lymph vessels for circulation. The skin contains about 5% of all of the blood and is one of the ways that it is directly connected to every other organ in the body. The skin also secures the sebaceous glands. Sebaceous glands secrete the body's natural oils called sebum. Sebum lubricates and waterproofs the skin. The proper amount of it moisturizes your skin giving it a smooth youthful appearance. Too little of it and your skin looks dry; too much of it and your skin looks oily; excessive amounts of it and you become prone to acne.

In addition to the above contents, approximately 75% of the dermis is made up of collagen, while 4% is elastin. These key fibers prop up the outer skin while giving it its strength and elasticity.

Collagen is made up of long chains of amino acids. Amino acids are organic compounds made up of carbon, oxygen, hydrogen and nitrogen to form various proteins. There can be as many as 50 variations of amino acids in the collagen. The most common and vital Collagen amino acids are L-lysine, L-glycine and L-proline. Collagen literally has the tensile strength of steel, yet it is supple. This is what gives your skin its fullness and structural strength. The more collagen the more wrinkle free and smoother the skin. Collagen is the skin's foundation fiber. A strong foundation ensures a solid skin. Collagen acts as a filter to reduce penetration of toxic microorganisms into the body. Our bodies produce collagen through a series of cells known as fiberblasts. As we age the fiberblasts have a much reduced capacity to produce more collagen. After age 21 that capacity is reduced by about 1% per year. As we lose collagen our skin not only loses firmness and smoothness, it also loses thickness. We start to see wrinkles and skin transparency, the signs of aging.

Another critical protein needed for youthful skin is elastin. Many people have heard about collagen, not as many have heard about elastin. Elastin, like collagen, is made up of amino acids. Where collagen offers strength and suppleness to the skin, elastin offers elasticity and bounce back. Elastin is primarily composed of the amino acids L-glycine, L-valine, L-alanine, and L-proline. Elastin is produced the same way as Collagen via the connective tissue cells known as fiberblasts. In the case of elastin the fiberblasts will secret a soluble molecule called tropoelastin which it then transforms into elastin after it goes thru a catalytic reaction with the body enzyme lysyl oxidose.

It should be noted that no matter what you put on or in your body, if you don't have or provide the proper enzymes to convert it so that it can properly integrate into your cells than it will just pass through and do nothing or possibly even do some harm. This is true of nutrients and vitamins. We will talk about this in more detail in a later chapter.

When we are younger if we squeeze our skin together and then release it, the skin goes back to its original shape virtually instantly. That is due to the elastin content. It is harder for wrinkles to form when the skin has elasticity. Just like a rubber band, when it is new no matter how you distort it or twist it or stretch it, the band will always come back to its original smooth shape. When the rubber becomes old and dried out it distorts and loses its snap back. The same is true for your skin when the elastin content either dries out or degrades. The rules that apply to collagen also apply to elastin, the older we get, the less we produce. That is the reason as we age instead of an instant bounce back the skin takes longer and longer to go back to its original shape and wrinkles can more easily form.

Below the dermis is the hypodermis. This is also referred to as the subcutaneous layer of skin. It is comprised mainly of adipose. Adipose is a fatty tissue that serves to store fat soluble vitamins such as A, D, E, and K. This fat cushions the body to reduce damage from an impact. It also insulates the body from severe weather or temperature and maybe most importantly its high vitamin content is the source of fuel to keep the rest of the body operating properly and efficiently. Without fuel the body can't produce collagen and elastin. Without collagen and elastin, the skin ages.

As we age the fatty tissue in the hypodermis starts to atrophy. This is usually due to a loss of proper nutrition. In fact, this lack of nutrition coupled with external harmful practices eventually causes atrophy to affect all of the layers of the skin along with other organs.

When we are younger our body cells are fresh and unscarred. They are more energetic and will produce and reproduce at a rapid rate even if they are not externally fueled up properly. There is no lack of internal positive energy in our bodies at a younger age which can somewhat compensate for a lack of healthy external nutrition. However, as we age we expose our bodies to a combination of all or part of the following: exposure to UV rays, food containing damaging ingredients going in our bodies, skin and personal care products with bad chemicals going on our bodies, oxidation, too many drugs, lack of enough exercise, stress, bad chemicals we put on our skin, not enough sleep, and drinking or smoking too much. These elements are constantly accumulating in our body and can eventually reach a high enough level that they start to wear down and break down our skin along with our body.

But that can be stopped and even reversed if we change course and do those things that revitalize and reinvigorate those ten trillion cells in our bodies. I know without question that we do not have to age at the rapid rate we have come to accept. The aging process can definitely be slowed down if we do the right things. The earlier we start the more effective the results.

Exercising and enough sleep will have positive effects. Making sure what we put in and on our body is good for our body is critical.

We need to supplement our skin with external, healthy, non toxic nutritional sources. If we do that our skin will maintain a youthful appearance far beyond its years. That is true for all of our organs as well.

Collagen and elastin losses can be slowed down. It can even be rebuilt. This will keep our skin firm and elastic and wrinkle resistant. We will show how to do this in the proceeding chapters. We will also explain why many of the methods touted in ads are not the way to do that.

Another requirement to keep the skin youthful looking is to protect it from the sun's rays. Most of the so called age or liver spots on our skin are not either from our liver or our age, it is because of UV ray damage from the sun. A lot of that occurs because the mislabeling and misconceptions about sunscreens are rampant around the world. They are especially bad in the United States, maybe more so than anywhere else in the world. In fact, many of the sunscreens actually aid the damaging of our skin and even induce skin cancer.

I know that we are constantly deluged with information and statements and claims about how to keep the skin healthy or how to repair damaged skin. This comes to us from the web, from television ads including infomercials, from magazines supposedly devoted to beauty do's and don'ts.

How many times have you been impressed with before and after photos showing wrinkles virtually disappearing in seconds? Let me just say that no matter how many times the ad promoter or voice over says the product shown is safe or natural or healthy – you should be wary. The terms "natural" or "organic" or "safe" by themselves usually define nothing and can be very misleading. It is virtually never safe or natural or healthy to alter the skin in a matter of moments. You may be able to cover up a problem but there are usually side effects that will uncover themselves over time.

If you truly want to diminish wrinkles or other skin defects there are healthy ways to do that, but just like losing weight, to do it right and keep it right without side effects will usually take some time. Not inordinate amounts of time, but certainly more than an hour or a day. It is the purpose of this book to show you those ways in the chapters that follow.

I also understand that the hardest thing for people to accept is change. We get caught up in what we are doing and have been doing for years and sometimes it takes an Act of Congress for us to change and even that may not do it. I spent over 30 years putting on motivational talks in the chemical processing industry trying to get people to change and improve upon what they were doing. The resistance to change was overwhelming even when it was unquestionably obvious. The larger the company the harder it was to get people within that company to throw out years of habits and fight all the layers of upper management to make those changes. After all, "rocking the boat" can be a perilous journey. It is that same mentality in beauty care corporations that resists the changes and maintains the same paradigms: the larger the company the more of the same. Even when they come out with something "new" they tend to follow the same path as the "old": chemicals on top of chemicals, toxins on top of toxins.

I do believe that when it comes to one's health most people will make the change away from the bad and towards the good. The problem has been that the industry has been so adept in hiding the facts that people do not have the tools or the knowledge to make the changes necessary. Hopefully the following chapters will not only give you the tools and knowledge but also the depth of understanding so that you can follow a path to keep your skin and body youthful appearing and healthy at the same time.

CHAPTER SIX
AGRICULTURE HARMS THE SKIN

SYNTHETICS ARE SINFUL

It is not the purpose of this book to analyze, define or propose what to put in the body. However, what we put in our body does affect our skin and many ingredients used to make skin care products are derived from agricultural sources and processes. It is sad but true, the food of today is grown with many chemicals and processed with even more chemicals that usually are not good for you.

Read the ingredient list on the foods you buy and look them up on websites to get at least some minimum understanding of what they may be doing to your body. Certainly it should concern you when you see that 40 or 50 ingredients were used to make those packaged foods and half of the ingredients have names 20 letters long.

Probably one of the most devastating actions that compromised the food industry occurred in the early 1990's with the acceptance of GMO's (Genetically Modified Organism's) by the World Health Organization (WHO), the Federal Drug Administration (FDA), the Environmental Protection Agency (EPA) and the United States Department of Agriculture (USDA).

Food was taken out of the hands of Mother Nature and put into the labs of chemical companies. The amount of testing done to determine how safe GMO's were was minimal at best and performed by the companies producing the seeds and chemicals to grow GMO's.

The hype was that farmers could produce a lot more crops on the same amount of land with a huge reduction in crop loss due to insects or airborne bacteria. Yes, that was true. However, they did not really tout or discuss one important caveat. In order for this to be achieved, seeds would have to be altered so that the plants they grew would be more resistant to damage from pesticide infusion. In other words, the plants could resist dying from the huge amounts of pesticides and insecticides that would be sprayed on them so that devouring insects and bacteria could not survive in that same space.

That meant more toxins, up to 10 times more toxins, could be sprayed on our food sources and animal feeds then what is used in non GMO's. What is even more disconcerting is that most GMO's, whether they be fruits, vegetables, ingredients in packaged foods or used as feed for beef, poultry or fish, especially in the USA, do not have to be disclosed as being GMO's. Certain Senators tried to pass through the DARK Act in 2016. DARK stands for Denying Americans the Right to Know what was in their food. Again, rather than protecting Americans, some members of the government preferred to protect toxic chemical manufacturers. Thank God it was defeated in March of 2016. Unfortunately, when money talks, morality walks. I have no doubt it will be tried again. Hopefully by the time you are reading this book the laws will have been changed to demand that companies must define all GMO ingredients and individual fruits and vegetables as such. Many of those chemicals are hidden from you. I would strongly suggest that you take the time to understand the food you eat and the supplements you take. The true nutrient value of our food is far below what it was 50 years ago and the toxin level is far above.

What is amazing is that the experts making up the President's Cancer Panel stated on page 43 of their May 2010 Report the following:

*"**Pesticides (Insecticides, Herbicides, and Fungicides).** Nearly 1,400 pesticides have been registered (i.e., approved) by the Environmental Protection Agency (EPA) for agricultural and non-agricultural use. Exposure to these chemicals has been linked to brain/central nervous system (CNS), breast, colon, lung, ovarian (female spouses), pancreatic, kidney, testicular, and stomach cancers, as well as Hodgkin and non-Hodgkin lymphoma, multiple myeloma, and soft tissue sarcoma.147 Pesticide-exposed farmers, pesticide applicators, crop duster pilots, and manufacturers also have been found to have elevated rates of prostate cancer, melanoma, other skin cancers, and cancer of the lip."*

In a letter to the President inserted in the beginning of that same report made the following observation:

*"**Most** (people) **also are unaware that children are far more vulnerable to environmental toxins and radiation than adults.**"*

One of the reasons that toxins are more dangerous to children then they are to adults is because a child's metabolism operates differently than an adult which means toxins remain longer in a child's body thereby doing more damage.

Relative to their body weight, children eat, breathe, and drink more than adults do. So children take in higher concentrations of any toxins in their food, water, or air. As organs develop, they are more likely to be damaged by exposure to toxins. The methods the body uses to remove toxins from bodies of adults are not fully developed in children.

All of this was stated and understood from the President on down in 2010, yet no changes or protections by any government agency have been initiated of any consequence in the United States.

The rest of the world has done something about it. Over 30 countries, including the entire European Union, have banned all or a major portion of crops harvested using GMO technology. Many of those same countries have banned the importing of USA GMO harvested products. Almost 90% of the corn grown in the USA is a GMO product and its importation is completely banned by both China and Russia.

There are approximately 14,000 chemicals used in processing food in addition to the 1400 pesticides used in growing food. Neither the FDA nor the EPA does their own testing of any of these chemicals, but as stated in chapter 1, they rely on data provided by the manufacturer of these chemicals to let them know how safe the product is to humans and animals. This is scary to say the least.

Many of those same chemicals plus 70,000 more are used in the Beauty Care Industry. That is even scarier.

The beauty industry advertises many of their products as being "natural" or "petroleum free". Those words ring hollow. In today's world that does not mean it is toxic free even if so stated. If the ingredient is derived from a vegetable source, it could be just as toxic as if it was derived from a petroleum source.

The five major GMO crops in the USA are Canola, Corn, Cottonseed, Soy, and Sugar Beets. Canola and Corn are a major source of vegetable oils. Here is where we can see that many of the toxicity problems associated with food also apply to skin care products.

For example, Glycerol is a major ingredient in thousands of skin care products and is derived from vegetable oils. Glycerol serves as a humectant. Humectants in skin care products perform two functions, one is to get water into the skin and two is to allow other chemicals to be driven into the skin. Neither of these actions is generally good for the skin because sometimes the water is pulled out of deeper layers in the skin where it is needed. In addition, the skin is being negatively altered thereby allowing toxins in the skin care product to drive deeper down into the skin layers eventually entering and harming other organs.

Glycerol is usually defined in the ingredients list as vegetable or vegetarian sourced as if that is a good thing. However, in more cases than not they are GMO based which is toxic. As people become more aware of the negative aspects of glycerol the skin care companies are listing the ingredient by many different names including 1, 2, 3-PROPANETRIOL; 1, 2, 3-TRIHYDROXYPROPANE; 1, 2, 3PROPANETRIOL; CONCENTRATED GLYCERIN; GLYCERINE; GLYCEROL; GLYCYL ALCOHOL; 1,2,3-PROPANETRIOL; 1, 2, 3-TRIHYDROXYPROPANE; 90 TECHNICAL GLYCERINE; CITIFLUOR AF 2.

This is only one example of where hundreds of so called natural products are hyped as being good for you when in reality they are not.

The beauty industry, like the food industry has spent millions of dollars to prevent the US government from forcing them to list ingredients as being GMO. This keeps it hidden from the public to the public's detriment and allows products to be shipped around the world skirting the GMO issues in other parts of the world. This action results in not letting consumers know what is going in their body or on their body. This takes away the individuals ability to choose or be able to make knowledgeable decisions to protect themselves. It should not be allowed to continue.

A group of people, in search of healthy food alternatives have become Vegetarians. There is an old joke that states "The word Vegetarian comes from an old Indian word meaning – me no hunt so well." But jokes aside, with today's farming methods it may not be as healthy of an alternative as first thought.

Even when you choose Organic food products, remember that Organic farming only means that no synthetic pesticides can be used on the crops. Instead, in many cases the Organic farmer will use a pesticide consisting of copper sulfate. Copper sulfates are not as effective in fighting bacterium, fungi or insect infestation so they tend to be applied more often than synthetic pesticides. A high buildup of copper sulfate on the fruit is not good for the human body either. Remember, if it is a pesticide it has to have the capability to kill. Copper sulfate applied directly to the body is a toxin and can be just as harmful as a synthetic pesticide.

If the farmer is conscientious and cognizant that over usage of copper sulfates is toxic, then the organic fruit is safer than the non-organic fruit. Just be aware that may not always be the case.

CHAPTER SEVEN
WOMEN VS MEN VS
TOXINS IN SKIN CARE

A major concern of mine is the different effects toxins can have on women verses men. Without question women purchase and use many more skin care products than men. This unto itself opens women up to higher amounts of toxin intake from beauty products.

But there is a second and more disconcerting issue also. Toxins are more likely to have more of a detrimental effect on a woman as opposed to a man due to the physiological differences between the two sexes.

Women overall have a more complex body than men. The higher the complexity of any functioning instrument increases the chances of it getting damaged. In addition, women have a less acidic stomach than men which means it can take longer to break down toxins when ingested. Men's kidneys tend to filter out toxins faster than a women's kidney therefore giving toxins more time to do more damage in a women's body. The liver also detoxifies chemicals and metabolizes drugs. Women's livers work slower then men's livers and therefore toxins tend to remain at their full damaging effect for longer periods of time than they do in men. Women have more body fat than men which means when they are exposed to toxins, especially those topically applied via skin care products, the toxins tend to linger longer in the fat tissue and therefore can have a more toxic effect on the body.

On July 14, 2014 the Scientific American Journal published an article showing how drugs affect men and women differently. It was written by Roni Jacobson which stated the following:

From animal studies to clinical trials, drugs are often tested on males only. Yet eight out of 10 drugs pulled from the market by the FDA between 1997 and 2001 posed greater health risks for women than men, according to a government report. This testing bias can be unwitting or intentional—many clinical trials exclude women because their different hormones are considered a "confounding variable." Pregnant women also typically do not take part in clinical trials for safety reasons, but mounting evidence suggests that their hormonal changes can alter the effects of certain drugs. For example, a study last year found that pregnant women with bipolar disorder require higher doses of the drug Lamictal to control their depression. In addition, medications taken only by women, such as birth-control pills, may interact with psychotropic medications with unknown consequences. The FDA recently announced that it would step up its effort to account for sex differences in clinical trials.

In simple terms, women are much more prone to toxic degradation then men. Yet, because of all the cosmetics including mascara, rouge, lip stick, make up, facial cleansers, moisturizers, plus hair color dyes, under arm deodorants, perfumes and eye lash thickeners: women put on as much as 200 more toxic chemicals on their bodies than men do every single day.

The renowned International Dermal Institute states the following on their website:

Skin Thickness

We know that the thickness of the skin varies with the location, age and sex of the individual. Additionally, androgens (i.e. testosterone), which cause an increase in skin thickness, accounts for why a man's skin is about 25 percent thicker than that of a woman's. A man's skin also thins gradually with age, whereas the thickness of a woman's skin remains constant until about the age of fifty. After menopause, her skin will thin significantly, which will continue as she ages.

Collagen Density

Regardless of age, men have a higher collagen density than women; this is the ratio of collagen to the thickness of the skin. Researchers believe that the higher collagen density accounts for why women appear to age faster than men of the same age. When considering intrinsic (genetically-programmed) aging of the skin, it has been said that women are about 15 years older than men of the same age. Of course, the role of daylight exposure in skin aging, combined with the fact that men do not use sunscreen as often as women, may account for why we do not readily notice. Extrinsic aging from UV radiation can add years to a man's skin and negate the benefit of slower intrinsic aging.

Loss of Collagen

The physical signs of aging in adults, such as wrinkles and laxity to the tissue, are closely related to the collagen content of the skin. Both men and women lose about one percent of their collagen per year after their 30th birthday. For women, however, this escalates significantly in the first five years after menopause then slows down to a loss of two percent per year.

Collagen has two critical functions. One of them is to firm up the outer skin. So yes, a thinner collagen layer means less firm skin and eventually more wrinkles. But there is a second function of collagen as discussed earlier. The tightness and layered thickness of the collagen cells also serves to keep out and filter out the passage of liquid or airborne molecules such as bacteria from the epidermis level of the skin into the dermis and beyond. With a thinner collagen layer in women's skin it allows for the potential of more toxins in skin care products being put on the body to pass through not only into the dermis but into the hypodermis below and eventually the blood stream. This means toxins from the outside can more easily make it into all the organs in a women's body as compared to the potential of doing the same in a man's body.

Certainly skin care manufacturers know this to be true and if they truly were concerned with protecting their customers, especially their female customers they would be using a lot less chemicals, especially toxic chemicals in their products then they are presently doing.

Certainly we are all aware that the amount of toxins in a single jar of any skin care product is not enough to cause major, or even minor health problems. In fact, this is the justification that the American Chemical Council (ACC) gives to the FDA, EPA and USDA as to why it is safe to put known toxic chemicals into skin care products. Remember it is much less expensive to fill jars with chemicals then it is to fill them with organic non GMO ingredients. Also remember that virtually all the testing to study the effects of chemicals on the human body is done by this same organization, the ACC. As we had stated in Chapter One, the ACC is owned and controlled by the same chemical companies that make those toxic chemicals. Of course they are going to "prove" that small amounts won't hurt anyone.

That may be true; a small amount of some toxins may not always be fatal. However, they are always bioaccumulative. To understand what bioaccumulative means let's reference back to cigarette smoking. Nobody gets lung cancer after smoking just one cigarette. It's the accumulation of tar and nicotine after years of usage that will do you in. The same is true of toxin accumulation from beauty products after years of usage.

In many cases, the body has no way of cleaning out those toxins going into your body through your skin. Your kidneys may clean out the portion of chemicals getting into your bloodstream. However, that is no guarantee either. The kidneys cannot clean up or remove many chemicals. This is especially true in the case of petroleum based chemicals. A lot of the toxins end up in the fat layers of the hypodermis. Not only do they bioaccumulate there, eventually attacking or destroying the good cells in that layer, but they also slow down or prevent the **<u>adipose</u>** cells in the hypodermis layer from performing their function of passing healthy nutrients into the rest of the body.

Adipose cells provide the nutrients to the upper cells in the skin to generate new cells for the replacement of the dying cells on the surface of the skin. It also is the source of hormones and energy needed for the entire endocrine system in the body. Adipose fiber contains cells vital to your immunity system; it is the major source of healthy energy and fuel for the entire body. A lot of stem cell research is centered on the adipose cells. It is felt if we can reproduce adipose cells and inject them into the body we can not only reduce the aging process, but can eliminate many diseases and increase the age to which we healthily live well beyond the 100 year mark. Bioaccumulation of toxins can interfere with that critical process.

CHAPTER EIGHT
PLUMP & PLUG VS
RENEW & REPAIR

We have all seen those ads where they either show before and after pictures, or in the case of videos they show a close up of a face that has wrinkles and then the wrinkles disappear within 15 minutes or less after applying the new miracle cream that is being advertised. In order to give it authenticity the spokesperson is either one of the most beautiful women on earth without a single flaw on her skin or they have a man in doctor's garb saying he either recommends the product or in the alternative, he has spent the last 15 years working on developing a non medical instant wrinkle eliminator cream and this is it.

A lot of these commercials are done as infomercials and shown on TV in the wee hours of the night preying on viewers who may be somewhat tired and therefore might not be in as a discerning mode as they would be at a normal hour. Thus, acceptance of the miracle cream becomes more plausible. But then again many ads are shown all during the day touting the cure is here.

How many times do we buy into the hype therefore buying the product only to discover in most, if not all cases, the product "ain't" quite what was advertised.

First of all, let me state that there are ways to replenish and restore your skin. Maybe you can't take off 20 years in twenty minutes, but I believe taking off a number of years in ten weeks is more than possible. But before we talk about the right way to do it, let's talk about the wrong way, the unhealthy way that is practiced by a majority of the skin care companies.

Yes, in the advertisements for skin care products you see terms like "moisturizing" or "firming up the skin" or "collagen building" or "anti wrinkling/ anti ageing". These are great catch phrases, but in too many cases are misleading and untrue.

Almost 90% of the skin care products sold in the USA work via a very unhealthy plump and plug concept. In simple terms that refers to a technique where chemicals, especially water accumulating chemicals, are used that will drive beneath the surface of the skin and then swell up with water. As they swell up they **PLUMP** up the epidermis above. The more water and chemicals that can be driven underneath, the firmer and less wrinkled the outer skin appears. These water attracting chemicals, also known as humectants, normally evaporate out much too fast which means the skin will go right back to where it was before you put on your so called "anti aging moisturizer."

In order to lock in the water and water bearing chemicals under the skin for as long as possible another series of chemicals, known as occlusives, are added to the formula. These chemicals **PLUG** up the pores in order to slow down the evaporation process so that the chemicals and water won't immediately evaporate out and therefore keep your skin looking as firm and wrinkle free for as long as possible. The occlusives are also referred to as being comedogenic.

The quicker the chemicals can plump and plug, the quicker the moisturizer will "repair" the skin. Unfortunately, this is a short term solution with a long term health damaging and skin damaging result. A general rule of thumb is that the more expensive the skin care cream, the more the long term damage. The reason for that is if you are paying $50 or $100 per jar, you expect and demand results in the short term. The manufacturers know that. To get those results requires fast absorbing humectants and quick acting occlusives. In many cases the chemicals chosen are quicker acting, more expensive and more toxic.

You never want a skin care product that is comedogenic. If it doesn't say it is non comedogenic stay away from it. We will discuss this in more detail below.

In the chapter entitled "Agriculture Harms The Skin" we talked about Glycerol being a humectant and have defined humectants as a means to get water into and under the skin. It also has a second function which is to alter the skin configuration to allow other chemicals to be driven into the skin. Altering the skin to absorb chemicals is never a good thing. It minimizes the skins natural ability to keep out bad stuff. The water is being used to fill in for the loss or lack of collagen and elastin. Water however does not have the strength of collagen, nor the elasticity. Plumping with water may diminish some of the wrinkles, but the skin quickly reverts back as soon as the water evaporates out.

Let me expand upon the statements made above. People can use moisturizers all year around, but they tend to be most needed when the air is dry such as during the winters in the north, and during dry seasons in the South and South West. When the air is dry it actually pulls water out of the body which is one of the reasons that your outer skin tends to flake and buckle up, as in wrinkling. If you have a lot of humectants on or in your skin then the water will be drawn up from your own deeper skin layers, especially the hypodermis layer which depletes your natural water content and actually demoisturizes the skin and body rather than moisturizes. The hypodermis contains most of the nutrients and fiberblasts cells that fuels your skin to build up your collagen and elastin. Depleting it of water, especially water that may contain nutrients, slows down the collagen generation capability and actually is damaging the skin. This is the complete opposite of what you want to do. Once water gets into the humectant it will eventually vaporize out of the body along with the humectant carrier chemical.

Using occlusive chemicals that perform a comedogenic action to block your pores and slow down evaporation is truly dangerous.

The skin regulates the body temperature via sweating and absorption. The skin also rids your body of toxins and excess sebum buildup (Your body produces sebum in the sebaceous glands located beneath your hair follicles in the dermis layers. Sebum is the oil your body produces to lubricate, as well as waterproof your skin and hair). Too much sebum and you can induce acne and blackheads. along with several other skin disorders. Blocking the pores seriously inhibits the skin from doing its job. Temperature regulation is inhibited, Toxins and sebum builds up to damaging levels just below the epidermis.

Some of the more popular humectants used in skin care products are glycerin (which we discussed in the chapter entitled Getting Under Your Skin) and hyaluronic acid, AHAs, sodium PCA, urea, trumella extract, and dicyanamide.

The popular occlusives are mineral oil, petrolatum, lanolin, and dimethicone.

Most of these are not good for the skin or the body.

Let's look at the humectants first.

1- **Hyaluronic acid** is touted in skin care products as if it were a miracle additive. Hyaluronic acid is a naturally occurring substance in the human body. One of its properties is that it can hold up to 1000 times its own weight in water and thereby offers fantastic hydrating properties. The highest natural concentration of it in the body is found in the joints, skin cells, and the eyes. When injected it can help with osteoporosis and is approved by the FDA for injection into the eye during cataract operations to keep the eye moisturized. These are pharmaceutical grades.

Skin care products do not use a pharmaceutical grade of hyaluronic acid. Most of the grades used in skin care is derived from the combs of roosters. The many claims attributed to hyaluronic acid are based on the injected form of it. There is no evidence or testing done with Hyaluronic acid that supports the claim it helps the skin, builds up collagen or anything else, when it is applied topically via a skin care cream. It has a fairly large molecular structure size and as a result does not penetrate too far into the skin. For the most part it just lays on the surface and will easily wash off leaving no long term benefits for the end user. It may be good when injected, but it is virtually useless in a topical cream or serum other than a temporary water absorber.

2- **AHA stands for Alpha Hydroxy Acid**. They are nothing new and actually have been used as a beauty aid going back to Cleopatra. When used in concentrations higher than 4% they exfoliate the skin and carry away dead cells from the epidermis. They are also used in skin moisturizers at concentrations under 3%. and are the acids derived from food sources such as follows;
-glycolic acid from sugar cane
-lactic acid from milk
-malic acid from apples and pears
-citric acid from oranges and lemons
-tartaric acid from grapes

Glycolic and Lactic are the most used and have the most testing done with them. They serve as humectants but also seem to be able to reverse skin damage due to the sun's rays known as photoaging. However, they can cause skin irritation and as a complete paradox to their use, they are known to make the skin more susceptible to photoaging if you go in the sun with it on. It's kind of like, well let me help you get rid of the wrinkles that I am about to add to your skin. In fact, AHA's are one of those rare ingredients that the FDA has actually set up guidelines for, not rules, just guidelines. They state that in order to use AHA's safely they should only be used on the skin if you are using a strong sunscreen at the same time. I personally would recommend staying away from them in a skin cream. They may be listed in the ingredients list under the five acid names above or just by the term AHA.

3- **Sodium PCA** (PCA stands for pyroglutamic acid) is a naturally occurring agent in the human body. Besides being a humectant it is also a conditioner for skin and hair. It is not toxic unto itself. The one concern about it is that depending on the grade used it can contain impurities and under certain circumstances will form Nitrosamines which are extremely toxic.

4- **Urea**, depending on its chemical make up can be both a humectant and a preservative. It is basically derived from animal urine although synthetic forms of it exist. In most cases when it is used in a cosmetic product the complete definition of its chemical make up is not shown in the ingredients list. Depending on the form (Benzimidazole urea, diazolidinyl urea, imidazolidinyl urea or polyoxymethalene urea) it goes from mildly toxic to severely toxic. Most forms of it release formaldehyde into the body. Formaldehyde is a great preservative if you are already dead but not so good if you are still alive.

5- **Trumella** extract is actually derived from mushrooms. It is non toxic and is even used in certain Chinese recipes and medicines.

6- **Dicyanamid** can be both an eye and a skin irritant. It is usually added to a skin care product to enhance the water absorbing capabilities of other humectants in the formula, especially Urea.

The most popular occlusive, or pore pluggers, are the following:

Mineral oil
petrolatum
lanolin
dimethicone.

Another concept used by many skin care companies is to use what I refer to as the "miracle drug" of the week. Since there is virtually no government overseeing of skin care products many "claims" can be made without any legal consequences. For example, there are two popular ingredients added into skin care products with some spectacular marketing promises made about them.

Peptides

One of these "miracle" ingredients comes in various forms of Peptides. The Peptides are usually claimed by the manufacturer to have excellent collagen building and anti wrinkle capabilities. Peptides are basically molecules that contain anywhere from 2 to 50 variations of amino acid compounds. Anything over 50 variations of amino acid compounds in one molecule brings it away from the peptide classification and carries it into the protein classification. As people age they tend to lose collagen which is the foundation fiber under the outer skin giving it fullness and structural strength. Collagen is long chains of amino acids known as proteins that are bonded together by shorter chains of amino acids known as peptides. As you age and lose both collagen and peptides you lose the mass and firmness under the skin which gives it a smooth appearance and prevents wrinkling. What skin care companies tell us is if you topically apply peptides they will help build up your collagen and keep it bonded together just like younger skin. However, there is no proof of this actually being true. In fact, there are a lot of facts that indicate it is not true.

In order to reach your collagen layer you have to penetrate below the skin's epidermis outer layers and down to the skin's deeper layers including the underlying Dermis layer. There is a Skin Law known as the 500 Dalton rule which governs capability of deep penetration. In order to penetrate deep into the skin the molecular size of the ingredient must be smaller than 500 Daltons.

A Dalton is the definition of an atomic size diameter no greater than about 0.00000001 of a millimeter in diameter. Therefore 500 Daltons is 0.000005 millimeters or 0.00000002 inches in diameter. To put it in perspective, if the head of a pin is 1/8" in diameter, it would take well over 6 million Dalton size particles lined up side by side to reach across the head of a pin. Peptides are usually much larger than 500 Daltons in molecular size.

Even if this was not the case, Peptides are generally unstable compounds. Other ingredients in the skin care cream can break them apart before they ever hit the skin. If they do make it to the skin, the enzymes in the skin will generally destroy them also. The chances of a topically applied Peptide giving the skin any long term enhancement of Collagen is woefully low in reality.

At Replenish Plus we are using a more proven and long term approach to helping skin with topical creams and/or serums. Instead of the detrimental Plump and Plug Methodology, we use the Repair and Renew method. Your body has the ability to fix almost everything that goes wrong if it is given the tools and nutrients to accomplish its task.

We can stop the most destructive diseases with zero side effects, not by outside medicines, but by inside cell generation. It was back in the late 1700's that Small pox was running rampant throughout the world. It actually brought many of the combatants in the Colonial (soon to be USA) Army to their knees during the Revolutionary War with Britain. It also infected many in the British Army who brought it back to their Mother Land. It was this epidemic that created the pandemonium and need for a solution. Dr. Edward Jenner, was the man who would do just that and become the Father and inventor of Immunization procedures as a result.

Dr. Edward Jenner was born on May 17, 1749, in Berkeley, Gloucestershire, England and was the son of the Rev. Stephen Jenner, vicar of Berkeley. Edward was orphaned at age 5 and went to live with his older brother. At a very early age he became interested in Science and Medicine. When he got older he trained in London to complete his apprenticeship in Medicine. He was dismissed as a quack because of his belief that feeding the body the proper compounds so it could build up anti bodies to destroy small pox was the only solution. In 1796, after years of research he felt that if you injected the body with a serum containing Cow Pox from cows, the human body could generate enough anti bodies to fight off the very human form of Small Pox. With threats of being arrested and disbarred from the medical profession that is exactly what he did to a small child in danger of falling victim to Small Pox. Nine days later the child was not only cured, but became immune to Small Pox for the rest of his life. This was the beginning of immunization and vaccine medicine for many diseases in the future.

Repair and Renew is a direct result of that same thinking. Find the proper serum or cream, made up of natural vitamins and nutrients so that the body gets charged up and can manufacture the proper skin cells to replace and recharge the dying cell areas of the skin. It doesn't happen in a day, or even a week. But one can start seeing results in a month or two. As long as you keep feeding the body it will keep repairing itself. It is not a non-lasting quick fix with harmful side effects. Instead it is a long term maintainable solution with healthy attributes for both the skin and the body.

At Replenish Plus we use botanical oils that contain stable nutrients with small molecular structures. Another way of penetrating the skin is to use oil soluble ingredients as opposed to water soluble oils. Since we do not use any water in our formulations, virtually all our ingredients are oil soluble. Oil solubility means it serves as a penetration enhancer. This occurs because oil solubility coincides with it being more slippery and therefore able to slip between the skin cell cracks and penetrate deeper down into the layers of the skin even when it is larger than 500 Daltons in diameter. By feeding the skin with natural vitamins, bioflavonoids, nutrients and enzymes, we basically are giving the skin nutritional food. Food to the skin is like gas to the car. It powers up the skin cell engines so they can produce and form healthy new cells, collagen and elastin. This is what gives the skin a youthful appearance for the long term.

The right way to reduce wrinkles, reverse the signs of aging and maintain a healthy looking skin is to not just moisturize, but more importantly to nutritionlize. The plump and plug method discussed above has only short term benefits to the skin but very long term detriments to both the skin and the body.

If you feed the skin a "cocktail" of Mother Nature's vitamins, nutrients, bioflavonoids and enzymes then it is giving the skin a whole food fuel boost. Synthetic vitamins are ineffective at best, and harmful at worse. We will discuss this in more detail in following chapters. Let it be suffice to say at this point that in order to reduce wrinkles, detoxify your skin, firm up your skin and give it a youthful appearance takes time and a proper approach. Any company that says it can do all or any of the above in a matter of minutes or days is outright lying. They can give a short time appearance, but not a long term solution.

Robert E Rockwood

It is no secret what has to be done. You can't put a coat of paint on anything and have it last unless you refurbish and prepare the surface underneath. The skin is constantly losing skin cells. If you can feed the skin with the proper nutrients, or fuel, so it can regenerate new healthy cells to replace the dying cells then the skin will start to glow. If you can inject Mother Nature's vitamins into the skin so it can build up the lost Collagen and Elastin, then after a period of time your skin will become firmer and smoother.

CHAPTER NINE
WORDS WITHOUT MEANING

When it comes to the skin care industry, manufacturers will use words to describe their product in the way that they know their clientele are looking for. What they don't tell their clientele is that since skin care is such an unregulated industry most of the so called high end identifying terms have little or no meaning when applied to skin care products.

In Chapter One we showed that the terms "clinically proven", "dermatologist tested" or "doctor approved" means absolutely nothing.

Other terms that beauty companies love to tout are "hypoallergenic", "allergy tested" and "non-irritating". There are no firm requirements to meet to use these terms. All it means is that the manufacturer feels that their product is less likely than other company products to cause an allergic reaction. There are no guidelines, regulations or laws that obligates the manufacturer to "prove" what they claim. Sad, but true.

Now let's look at the term "Natural". This term has a zero definition in the skin care industry. It literally means nothing. If a company has only one natural ingredient it can call their product "Natural". It could be 95% chemicals containing one drop of some natural product and call itself natural. Then again what is a natural product? Water, Petroleum, Arsenic, Urine, Copper Sulfates, Sand, Animal Parts, Lead, Botanicals laden with pesticides are all considered "Natural' All are used in skin care products. Anything not considered synthesized is natural. That does not mean it is good for you.

The term that beauty care companies really love to use is "Organic" because they know everybody thinks "Organic" is safe, healthy and wonderful. Again, in the skin care unregulated industry, the term Organic is nebulous at best. The only government agency that makes any reference to the term "Organic" as used in the skin care industry is the USDA (United States Department of Agriculture). Their regulations are loose at best.

USDA regulations for "Cosmetics, Body Care Products and Personal Care Products states the following:

1- *The FDA does not define or regulate the term "organic" as it applies to cosmetics, body care, or personal care products.*
2- *The USDA can only define the term "organic" as it pertains to agricultural products. No minerals, chemicals or animal products can have a USDA organic classification.*
3- *There are only two ways that a beauty care company can display the USDA Organic Seal on their product.*
   a- *The USDA Organic Seal and the term "100 Percent Organic" can only be used if the product contains only organically produced ingredients excluding water and salt. (This means the producer can put up to 90% water and salt in the jar and still call it 100% Organic)*
   b- *The USDA Organic Seal and the term "Organic" can be used if the product contains at least 95% organically produced ingredients excluding water and salt. (Again this means that a company can put up to 90% water and salt in the jar along with 5% of any nonagricultural ingredient and still call their product Organic)*

4- *A company cannot use the USDA Organic Seal but can use the term "Made With Organic Ingredients" if the product contains at least 70% organic ingredients excluding water and salt. The label must be able to display at least three organic ingredients. (Once again 90% of the product can be made up of water, salt and inorganic ingredients, including toxins, yet, still call their product "Made With Organic ingredients).*

The above are the only USDA definitions for Organic Beauty Products. If the USDA Seal is on the jar at least you can be confident that there are no toxins in the jar but it doesn't tell you anything about the amount of true organic products in the jar. You could have nothing more than a jar filled up with water and salt and a little tiny amount of some organic ingredient. If it says "Made With Organic Ingredients" you may have a whole bunch of water, salt and toxins in the jar.

But even worse than that is the loop hole statement in the USDA regulations for beauty products which is the following:

However:
- *USDA has no authority over the production and labeling of cosmetics, body care products, and personal care products that are not made up of agricultural ingredients, or do not make any claims to meeting USDA organic standards.*

- *Cosmetics, body care products, and personal care products may be certified to other, private standards and be marketed to those private standards in the United States. These standards might include foreign organic standards, eco-labels, earth friendly, etc.*
  The USDA does not regulate these labels at this time.

In other words, the USDA is saying as long as the product makes no reference to the USDA anywhere on the jar the company is free to use the word "Organic" no matter what is in the jar. **<u>Buyer Beware</u>**.

Another labeling loophole used by skin care companies to disguise where certain ingredients actually fall on a descending order list is to do two things that leave the enduser in the dark. One thing is to use the term "active ingredients" and "other ingredients". Under this system if a skin care company wants to claim that "organic rosehip oil" stimulates anti wrinkling and therefore is an active ingredient they can list it at the top of the ingredient list under a title that says "active ingredients" This way even if it comprises less than 2% of the formula it sits at the top of the listing. They can put more than one ingredient under the active ingredient title. Then underneath that listing they put the title "other ingredients" and list the remaining ingredients in descending order. The customer sees a clean expensive ingredient under active ingredients at the top and assumes it is the number one ingredient even though in reality it may be number 25.

Another "trick" is to use the words "proprietary blend". This way the manufacturer can list a whole bunch of ingredients under this title in any order it desires. By adding up the weight of all the ingredients in the so called "proprietary blend" it appears that this comprises a major portion of the cream yet says nothing about what the individual volume of each ingredient really is.

A truly masterful marketing trick is to give the product a name like "Organic Mango Cream". Since this is only a product name and is thereby under zero regulations, it can have nothing to do with the actual product or formulation. There does not have to be any organic ingredients in the jar or even any Mango. It could be totally inorganic and lacking even a single drop of Mango.

The point of all this? Always read the ingredient list. See how many ingredients are listed as organic. If the product name includes a certain ingredient name, check the ingredient listing to see if it is actually shown in the listing at all, and if it shown where does it fall on the listing. If it is towards the bottom there is not much in there at all.

As mentioned in Chapter One, a marketing ploy used by skin care companies is when they market a new product as containing an exclusive proprietary blend which contains rare rain forest extracts which will remove wrinkles in 15 minutes. They then give this new miracle wrinkle remover blend an exotic name like Kosmonificient and show it being used on a model whose wrinkles disappear in minutes. Usually when this is done, Kosmonificient contains an itsy bitsy drop or two of some exotic rain forest plant sap that may or may not have anything to do with removing wrinkles. Remember, there are no FDA regulations concerning claims made about resolving surface cosmetic issues like wrinkles. In reality, Kosmonificient is then formulated with up to 95% of some toxic chemical plasticizer which when it hits the skin actually deforms the skin and makes the wrinkles disappear. Of course, the wrinkle disappearance only last as long as the plasticizer is on your skin. Wash it off and so comes back the wrinkles and some skin damage from the toxic chemical being used. The brilliance of this type of marketing is they don't have to list the chemical they are using because it is part of the trademarked Kosmonificient proprietary blend.

One other area where words are used that hide the truth is regarding where the product is manufactured. Most people in the USA feel comfortable with products made in the USA, Canada, Japan, Australia, New Zealand or anywhere in Europe. It is rightfully understood that these countries generally abide to high manufacturing and quality control guidelines.

It is just as well believed, and in too many cases true, that many countries in Asia such as China and Thailand, along with third world countries like the Philippines and Indonesia do not maintain high standards in many of their plants.

Companies like to avoid denoting that their skin care product is manufactured in China, especially if it is marketed as a high priced exclusive brand.

The Federal Trade Commission (FTA) is the government agency which mandates the terms that can be put on a label to identify where the product is manufactured. When it comes to skin care or beauty products the regulations are loose at best. The FTA regulations reads as follows:

U.S. content __must be disclosed__ on automobiles and textile, wool, and fur products. There's no law that requires most other products sold in the U.S. to be marked or labeled Made in USA or have any other disclosure about their amount of U.S. content.

That regulation leaves a vast loop hole for any companies other than automobile and clothing manufacturers who want to avoid the "Made in China" revelation. Obviously that loop hole is used by some skin care companies.

The company may choose to not put any reference to where the product is made or where the ingredients are sourced from.

If they want to make you think it is made in a top tier country, they may include terms like "Distributed by" or "Made for" or "Bottled by" followed by the name of a company with an address in a top tier country. However, those terms tell you nothing as to where it is actually manufactured.

Any reliable, credible company will display a term that says "Made in America" or "Made in (Country of Origin)".

This is important to know. Skin care products are going to go in your skin and into your body regardless of claims otherwise. It is as intrusive to the body as food. You do not want to put products on your body that have been made in low quality locations that may contain containments not listed on the jar but infused into the product due to a dirty manufacturing environment.

If the product does not specify where it was made, then avoid using it on your skin. If it is specified but made in countries not known for keeping high quality standards, then I would still advise not putting it on your skin or body.

CHAPTER TEN
WATER – THE MOST TOXIC CHEMICAL OF ALL

How can water be a toxic chemical. Has the author (That of course would be yours truly) been sniffing too much of his beauty products and gone batty. Well, before I lose too much credibility let me explain one thing, it is not the water unto itself that is toxic, it is what has to be done to the water, by the water and for the water that makes it toxic.

First of all, let's explain why the water is in the skin care product. The answer is simple, water is cheap and the more a company puts into the jar the less of everything else has to go in and the higher the profits.

Close to 90% of all beauty products, especially skin care creams, have water as the number one ingredient. This is true whether the product cost $6 for 6 ounces in Walmart or if it costs $159 an ounce in a dermatologist office.

Lower cost products list it as the first ingredient and call it by its real name – water. However, as you go up the price scale the name may change from water to "purified water" to "aqua". Believe me, the name may change but the water is the same.

Some of the more devious skin care providers will avoid listing water as the number one ingredient and instead list Aloe Vera as the number one ingredient. In many cases this is water with a slight variation. The reason for that is they will use the most voluminous and least expensive form of the Aloe Vera inner gel layer which is 99% water.

There are three layers to each leave of the Aloe Vera plant. It is true that Aloe Vera is great for the skin and contains as many as 75 potentially active constituents including: vitamins, enzymes, minerals, nutrients and amino acids. However, what is not commonly known is that the leaves of the Aloe Vera are made up of three layers.

1- An inner clear gel layer which is 99% water
2- A hard latex layer
3- An outer rind

In order to really get the benefits that Aloe Vera has to offer as a topical agent for the skin you have to use a concentrated version where most of the water is eliminated and a combination of all three layers are properly constituted together.

When I use Aloe Vera in any of my formulas, I only use Aloe Vera concentrate and define it as such in my ingredient list. If the skin care ingredient list on the product you are using only defines it as Aloe Vera or Aloe Vera Leaf you can be pretty sure it is basically water with a 1% or less ineffective amounts of nutrients.

The skin care companies don't want to say they are using water or Aloe Vera water in order to cut their costs. Instead they put a spin on it. I talk to people selling skin care products, from sales staff in stores or spas to dermatologists and aestheticians in skin centers to find out what their skin care supplier has "taught" them to believe why water is in the product. I am always amazed at the reasons I am told why water is good in the product. Anywhere from "moisturizing" to "revitalizing" to "carrying other ingredients into the skin" to "cutting down on the oily feel of a cream".

Let me repeat one thing here – the only reason, and I do mean the only reason water is put into a product is to reduce the cost of manufacturing. There is not a single solitary benefit to the end user by having water in a beauty product. However, there are numerous detrimental and harmful effects. If you see water as the first, second or even third ingredient listed on a skin care product you should never buy it. Certainly you should never put it on your body.

I don't care who told you it is ok or good to use a water filled skin care or beauty product. They either don't know what they are talking about and/or they just want to sell you a product and don't give a damn about you.

Let's look at the truth and cut through the beauty care industry spin of lies and misleading statements.

No matter how dry your skin is, your body consist of between 65% and 75% water. That means if you weigh between 100 and 150 pounds, you consist of between 65 pounds and 110 pounds of water.

How much skin care moisturizing cream do you apply to your body each day? Let's go completely ridiculous and assume you have a 16 ounce jar of moisturizing cream and you use one jar up every week. That would mean you are putting on 2 ounces of cream every day. Even if 50% of the cream was water, that translates to adding 1 ounce (50% of 2 ounces) of water to your skin every day. There is no way that adding 1 ounce of water to a body that already contains a minimum of 1040 ounces (65 pounds X 16 ounces) of water is going to do anything. Realistically most skin creams are sold in 50 mm (1.7 oz) jars that are meant to last at least two weeks or more. That means you are only applying 1/10 of an ounce (1.7 oz divided by 14 days) daily to your body which already contains a minimum of 1040 oz of water. Believe me, that is doing absolutely nothing to help your skin or body.

In fact, if adding water to your body by applying it to the skin was going to do anything, you would see enormous improvements to your skin after every shower when you apply gallons of water to the surface of your skin. I don't remember ever hearing anybody coming out of the shower and saying to themselves "WOW, my skin looks and feels so young and it stays that way all day".

Adding water topically doesn't moisturize, it actually demoisturizes your skin and dries it out. I will explain more about that in a following paragraph.

Let us first explain why water in a skincare product is toxic. When water is listed as the number one ingredient it usually means that between 50% and 75% of the jar you just paid good money for is nothing more than water. Now here lies the problem. It is not the water itself that is toxic, it is the processing required for the water that turns it toxic. Three processes has to be performed on water in order to keep it in solution:

1- Water is runny and has to be thickened up otherwise the skin care cream is too liquidly.
2- Bacteria will form in water especially once it is exposed to the atmosphere. That means a preservative has to be added.
3- Water does not mix with oil. Oil always exist in a skin cream which means the water has to be chemically altered, known as emulsification, so it can mix with the oils in the formula.

Increasing the texture of the water is accomplished by adding a thickening agent. It should be noted that thickening agents are considered processing fluids. Processing fluids are exempt from being listed under the ingredient label. These are the so called "hidden ingredients" that we will be talking about in a future chapter. In some cases they may be listed but in most cases they are not. This again is one of those buyer beware situations. If water is in the ingredient list then some type of thickening agent is being used. Most of them are toxic which is why water adds toxicity to the skin care cream. There are various types of thickening agents used. Some of the more popular ones are listed below;

Polyacrylamide: A thickening ingredient for creams which is also used for manufacturing plastics and adhesives. This chemical is highly toxic and irritating to the skin. Causes central nervous system paralysis. Can be absorbed through unbroken skin.

Behenyl Alcohol: A thickening agent which is also used for manufacturing synthetic fabrics, insecticides and lubricants. It is a skin irritant.

Sodium Polyacrylate: A sodium salt of Polyacrylic Acid with concerns for organ system toxicity.

In order to keep the water bacteria free, it has to be preserved. There are a number of preserving agents but the ones that are most commonly used in skin care products fall into two categories:

formaldehyde releasers and parabens. Both of these families of chemicals are highly toxic.

For the same reason formaldehyde is used to preserve dead bodies, it is used for water preservation. The difference is if you are dead than the formaldehyde can't do you harm. However, if you are alive it is harmful to the immune system and highly carcinogenic, as well as a straight toxin to the body. That is why it is listed as a dangerous chemical by both OSHA and the EPA. In order to get around listing formaldehyde in the ingredient list, skin care companies use other names for it and in many cases use formaldehyde releasers which in my opinion is even worse than using formaldehyde.

Formaldehyde releasers do what they say; they release formaldehyde over time. In fact, the longer a jar of cream sits on the shelf the more formaldehyde is being released into the product. Than when you put it on your skin the moisture activates it even further so it produces formaldehyde going directly into the body.

The three common formaldehyde releasers are the following:

A) **Quaternium-15** which is a quaternary ammonium salt. The EU (European Union) has put a partial ban on its use and strictly limits the quantity that can be used. Not true for the USA. Use as much as you want and it's legal here.

B) **DMDM Hydantoin** is a fairly popular releaser. In addition to all the other formaldehyde issues, DMDM is also a skin irritant. This particular chemical is banned in Japan but can be used in the USA.

C) **Urea** compounds are probably the most popular formaldehyde generator. They are basically a family of preservatives that rely on the slow release of formaldehyde to keep products on the shelf longer. Besides being toxic and carcinogenic, they have also been identified as potential skin and tissue irritants. Your body produces Urea and rids itself of it as quickly as possible via the kidneys and into the urine. Commercially produced Urea is formulated using two raw materials, ammonia and carbon dioxide.

Parabens are Non Formaldehyde Preservatives

Parabens - The most popular preservatives used in the cosmetic industry are Parabens. Chemically, parabens are esters of p-hydroxybenzoic acid. The most common parabens used in cosmetic products are methylparaben, propylparaben, and butylparaben. Parabens are extremely toxic, hormonal disrupters and carcinogenic.

The European Union has found parabens to be so toxic that virtually all of them are banned from use in cosmetics sold in Europe. The Europeans basically only allow limited use of two parabens - Propylparaben and Butylparaben. These two cannot comprise more than 0.14% of total volume in any product.

However, in the USA all forms of parabens are allowed to be used in a skin care product in volumes up to 25% of the product. That is almost 200 times the amount allowed by law in Europe. Thankfully, very few US skin care products approach this volume but certainly volume percentages of 4 or 5% are not uncommon and is still 35 times higher than what Europe has found to be acceptable.

This is virtually an affront to women. Almost 90% of all breast cancer has been found to contain parabens. Maybe those parabens came from sources other than skin care products, but with that high of a percentage it is almost a crime not to ban its use in anything that coats or enters the body.

I have no question in my mind if these largely male owned cosmetic companies found out that 90% of all prostate or penile cancer were caused by parabens they would stop producing it in a heartbeat. To me, continuing to use parabens in their products is sexism at its worse.

As stated previously, if water is in the ingredient list, it must be emulsified in order to allow it to mix with the oils in the product. There are many different chemicals that will emulsify water. Virtually all of them are harmful and toxic. I will not try to list all of them but let me identify the most popular ones used by the skin care industry.

Diethanolamine (DEA): Used in cosmetics as an emulsifying agent. Considered to be highly toxic when used in industrial applications, and has been proven to cause cancer when applied to the skin of rats. And yet, this ingredient, and its derivatives, is permitted to be used in cosmetic products at limited levels. Derivative ingredients may appear as cocamide DEA or lauromide DEA. DEA can be found in over 600 cosmetic and personal care products.

Triethanolamine (TEA) is an emulsifier used in over 3000 skin care products in the USA. Yet it is listed as a toxin by OSHA and not allowed to get in contact with an employee who is working with it. Of course the skin care companies say it is all right to put it in their lotions because they are only using a small percentage in each product. My counter argument to that is if you knew I was giving you food that contained arsenic and I said it was only a small percentage of the recipe would you eat it Mr. Skin Care Company President?

Polyethylene Glycol (PEG) is another extremely popular emulsifier which is derived from the petrochemical gases ethylene and propylene. PEG's have been known to irritate sensitive or damaged skin and have been associated with kidney damage in animals. However, that is not the worst of it. According to a report in the International Journal of Toxicology by the Cosmetic Ingredient Review (CIR) committee, impurities found in various PEG compounds include ethylene oxide and 1,4-dioxane – both human carcinogens; polycyclic aromatic compounds (volatile chemicals that are also potentially cancer-causing); and heavy metals such as lead, iron, cobalt, nickel, cadmium, and arsenic. Both 1,4-dioxane and ethylene dioxide are listed as toxins on both the EPA and OSHA harmful chemical list.

However, the CIR (Chemical Industrial Review Board owned and funded by the cosmetics industry) concluded that PEGs are generally 'safe for use' in cosmetics but should 'not be used on damaged skin'. It is on this rather thin endorsement that PEGs continue to be used in skin care products. Let us not be fooled, their presence on the label indicates the product contains toxic and carcinogenic ingredients.

The conclusion to all of this is that if you see water or aloe vera as the first or second item listed under the ingredient list, you should probably stay away from that product and avoid the toxicity they generate by their presence.

Another item to be concerned about is that once water is emulsified it now has the capability of mixing with oil, that includes the natural oils your body produces to help keep your skin soft and silky. Once you ingest emulsified water into your skin, the water can and will mix with your natural oils. Most of this water will evaporate back out. Either it will do it shortly after sinking in to the skin, or if your skin care product is using a Plump and Plug formulation it will evaporate out once you have washed off the chemicals that are plugging your pores. This will have given even more time for the emulsified water to mix with your sebum and pull your healthy natural oils out of your body as the water evaporates and goes into the atmosphere.

The general rule of thumb is if you see water as the number one ingredient it probably represents between 55 and 65% of the contents. Another 25% of the contents more than likely consists of harmful chemicals needed to thicken, emulsify and preserve the water. That leaves you with maybe 20 to 25% of any ingredients that actually are good and helpful. Even that may be at question depending on how the manufacturer is approaching reducing ageing, wrinkles and dry skin. We will cover that in the following chapters.

In any case why would anyone want to buy a bottle of a skin care product that is 50% water, 25% chemicals used to alter the water and harm your skin, leaving only 25% of anything that may be arguably good for the skin.

At best you are wasting away your money, at worse you are wasting away your skin.

Take heart, there is a positive healthy alternative that will be discussed in the Mother Nature Chapter up ahead.

CHAPTER ELEVEN
WHAT ARE THOSE OTHER
CHEMICALS DOING

SYNTHETICS ARE SINFUL

Let me once again repeat, it is not my intent to provide you with a chemistry course and identify all the chemicals used by the Cosmetic Industry. After all, that entails tens of thousands of chemicals. I do want to identify those chemicals which I feel are the most harmful and are used the most frequently. This is not to cause a scare, but more importantly to make you aware.

Even if you don't retain or remember a single chemical that I denote in this book, that is okay. Here is what I do want you to remember: The natural reaction of your body is to reject and protect you from any chemical that is foreign to the natural aspects of Mother Nature. Look at the ingredient list of any product you are considering to buy and use. If the terms sound foreign to you, they are probably foreign to your body. Any questions about any ingredients, go to the website www.ewg.com (also reached via www.skindeep.com). EWG is the Environmental Working Group and they independently test and analyze thousands of skin care products and chemicals. Look up an ingredient to find out whether it is harmful or not.

Other than Mother Nature produced botanical plants, elements naturally produced by Mother Nature's creatures like beeswax and honey or basic elemental minerals like Zinc, Magnesium and Iron: your body will see everything else as an unwanted invasion. Maybe those chemicals will succeed in accomplishing some of its functions on the body, but the body will fight it hard enough to cause side effects.

How many times have we heard a medicine advertised on TV proudly espousing how it will cure some dreadful disease only to be followed by a much larger list of dreadful side effects? It's true for medicines, it's true for most skin care chemicals produced in a processing plant.

I have always felt that every time you put a chemical laden skin care product on your body you have just entered into chemical warfare with yourself.

We have identified a number of chemicals used for specific reasons by the Cosmetic Industry in previous chapters. Let us look at the other dirty chemicals used in cosmetics for various skin alterations.

I will preface the names of these chemicals with the following truth:

The faster that a company boasts in its advertisements it can resolve a skin care problem such as wrinkling – the more toxic the chemicals being used. You will get a short term result with a long term damage. Nothing alters the body quickly without a damaging side effect. In fact, in virtually all cases the short term result will quickly revert back to where it was, or worse, as soon as the chemical wears off or washes off.

That applies to everything you do to your body. You can lose weight by proper dieting and exercising OR you can take pills that bloat your stomach to cut down on hunger, increase your metabolism and/or act as a laxative to empty your intestines. The first method is healthy and maintainable for the rest of your life. The second method will shortly be rejected by your body and shorten your life.

In the Mother Nature chapter we will talk about what you should use to keep your skin youthful and your body healthy.

For right now let's talk about what not to use.

We have already listed a number of chemicals in previous chapters that are harmful and/or toxic. They have included the following:

Chapter 8

Hyaluronic acid
Alpha Hydroxy Acid
Sodium PCA
Urea
Cyanamid

Chapter 10

Polyacrylamide
Behenyl Alcohol:
Sodium Polyacrylate:
Quaternium-15
DMDM Hydantoin
Urea
Parabens
Diethanolamine (DEA)
Triethanolamine (TEA)
Polyethylene Glycol (PEG)

Skin Care companies use various chemicals to perform various actions:

Emolliants To Penetrate the Pores

One of the things that skin care companies want to do is drive their creams and serums into the skin as soon as possible. The reason for this is twofold: 1 – If they are using a "Plump and Plug" procedure they want the humectants under the skin ASAP. 2- Many women don't want their cream to feel oily. One way to accomplish this is by driving everything into the skin quickly.

This is done using a family of chemicals known as emollients or penetration enhancers. The problem with penetrants is that they are usually irritants by themselves. In addition, penetrants are not selective as to what they drive into the skin. They will drive all the toxins and carcinogens in the formula deeper into the skin along with everything else. Now the toxins are closer to your healthy underlayer of skin cells and organs in your body so they can more effectively damage them.

Disodium EDTA – This is a fairly harmless chemical unto itself, however it is a powerful penetrant that will carry virtually everything you put on your skin into your skin.

Synthetic Alcohols – A common penetrant made from petroleum byproducts. They tend to irritate the skin and because of their quick evaporation properties will dry out the epidermis.

Moisturizers to Condition/Lubricate the Skin

Mineral Oil – It is used in thousands of skin care products and promoted to be a moisturizing agent. This could not be further from the truth. In reality it is the absolute anti moisturizer. It absorbs very poorly which leaves it as a coating on top of the skin which blocks the pores and inhibits the bodies capability to function properly. It is phototoxic (i.e. makes the skin more prone to sunburn) and allergenic. It inhibits vitamins (A,D,E and K) from working properly. It is also used in a lot of lip balms. The most concerning problem is it contains the toxins and cancer producing agents PAH and 1,4-Dioxane (See Hidden Toxic Ingredients chapter).

Petrolatum – A semi solid petroleum jelly that has the same faults as mineral oil.

Cottonseed Oil – This is used as a skin conditioner. It is not the cottonseed oil that is the main problem it is what it contains. Depending how and where it is farmed it could be contaiminated with mercury, lead, arsenic and pesticides.

Making the Product Look, Smell and Feel Pretty

Fragrances/Parfum – This innocuous term is used to hide the largest number of toxins using a catch all phrase thet reveals nothing. Fragrances are the harbingers of as many as 200 toxins, carcinogens, irritants and hormonal disrupters in one blend. Stay away from products that list this as an ingredient.

Phthalates – These are Plasticizers used to smooth out the texture of creams and also make wrinkles disappear fast.

This product is banned in the EU and California for use in children's toys but present in many skin care products. It disrupts the endocrine system and causes cancer.

Coal Tar – Usually listed as a color plus a number. i.e. FD&C Red No. 6. This is an absolute known carcinogen which is banned in the EU (Europe) but allowed in the USA.

Vitamins to Give a Healthy Look to the Skin

Skin Care Product literature will proudly display how they are enhanced with Vitamins. Most users seek out those creams that have Vitamin C and/or Retinol A boldly highlighted on the jar. Once again the Beauty Care Producers have put a positive spin on a negative ingredient.

Yes, it is true that vitamins are good for the body. However, that comes with a caveat. Only Mother Nature can produce vitamins that are truly good for the body. When derived from Botanical Natural resources the vitamins are great.

When derived via processed synthetic chemicals they are usually harmful. This is the case for well over 90% of the vitamins supplied in skin care products. Let's look at two of them

Vitamin C – This vitamin is used to fight wrinkles because it helps to fight oxidation, promote skin cell immunity and increase skin elasticity. That is true when you get it from a natural source. However, skin care companies find it is much cheaper to manufacture synthetic ascorbic acid (Vitamin C) than it is to extract Vitamin C from plants or minerals. Although man made ascorbic acid replicates Vitamin C chemically it does not replicate the total compound including nutrients, bioflavonoids and enzymes. These three constituents are what makes natural Vitamin C work. Without them, Vitamin C actually works against you.

Synthetic Vitamin C when it hits the skin and becomes a free agent seeing moisture, temperature and bodily acids it usually decomposes within 45 minutes to an hour. At that point it is no longer working for you, it is working against you. It is no longer an anti-oxidant, it becomes an Oxidant attacking cells and breaking down the immune system. You are better off with no vitamin C if it is synthetic vitamin C.

Retinol A

Vitamin A (natural beta carotene) is excellent for fighting wrinkles and building the ability of skin cells to communicate properly and become normalized. Normal healthy cells are best equipped to stay healthy and fight the degradation causing wrinkles and vibrancy. Vitamin A has been shown to help fight many skin disorders including acne, eczema and psoriasis.

Once again the skin care companies will generally use a synthetic form of Vitamin A known as Retinol A. This form is extremely toxic and actually is rated at 9 on a scale of 1 (being the least toxic) to 10 (being the most toxic) on the EWG website. EWG states the following:

"Retinol is a potent form of synthetic vitamin A. Data from an FDA study indicate that retinoid ingredients may speed the development of skin tumors and lesions on sun-exposed skin. FDA, Norwegian and German health agencies have raised a concern that daily skin application of vitamin A creams may contribute to excessive vitamin A intake for pregnant women and other populations."

It has been found to be carcinogenic and because it may cause skin cell deaths it has been linked to cardiovascular disease.

Once again, skin care companies have chosen to use a toxic synthetic form of what would be a very helpful vitamin when applied in its natural form.

Stiffeners

These are chemicals that are used to raise the melting point of skin care creams.

Castor Oil Hydrogenated
Stearyl Alcohol
Cetyl Esters
Bees Wax

The beauty care industry in many cases adds stiffening agents to their creams so that it won't melt until it reaches 130 degrees F or higher. This is done for two reasons:

1- When the product is being shipped during the summer or to hot geographic areas they don't want the cream to melt while on route in a train or delivery truck.
2- They know that their customers may leave the product in a hot car during the summer and they want it to stay as a cream and not turn into a gooey liquid.

This is great for them from a shipping and marketing point of view. It is terrible for you, the customer. If the product does not fully melt until it reaches 130 degrees F, than that means it doesn't melt on or in your body. Your body temperature is at 98 degrees. Even if the surface of the skin is a little warmer in the summer, the undersurface is still at 98 degrees. When you put on a cream that doesn't melt until it reaches 130 F you are putting on a cream that will plug your pores (comedegenic) and shut down your body's ability to regulate its temperature or the ability to sweat out toxins. You do not want a cream unless it melts at 90 degrees or below. Anything else will wreak havoc with your internal regulation system.

Let me repeat what I have said over and over in this book because I believe without question that one should never use synthetic chemicals on their body. Certainly not on a regular basis.

Maybe you can't remember or learn the names of all the toxic chemicals but at least remember the handful of the more common ones listed above. Avoid putting those on your body whenever possible. A little arsenic doesn't kill everybody but it helps nobody. Why take the chance that you will be the one who is effected harshly?

CHAPTER TWELVE
THOSE DANGEROUS SECRET HIDDEN INGREDIENTS

SYNTHETICS ARE SINFUL

The FDA left a giant loop hole in the requirements stating that a cosmetic company had to list all of their ingredients considered part of the product formula in descending order somewhere on the packaging material. If another chemical is needed in order to manufacture a formula chemical, then that other chemical is considered a processing fluid and does not have to be listed. Another way chemicals become hidden is if they are a byproduct and formed during the processing method. These unlisted or hidden chemicals are usually the most toxic of all. Companies will go to extra lengths to classify these most dangerous of chemicals as processing chemicals rather than formulation chemicals and thereby eliminate the need to inform the end user they exist in their product.

IT SHOULD BE NOTED THAT HIDDEN INGREDIENTS ONLY EXIST WHEN SYNTHETIC CHEMICALS ARE USED IN THE FORMULATION OF A SKIN CARE PRODUCT. TRULY ORGANIC/NATURAL INGREDIENTS ARE NOT PROCESSED WITH TOXIC CHEMICALS

The most common hidden ingredients are the following:

Diethanolamine(DEA) – We had listed this chemical in Chapter 10 as an emulsifying agent. It is extremely toxic. However, it is used sparingly as an emulsifier and therefore only listed in a few ingredient lists. It is used as a processing agent to make numerous chemicals listed in skin care products. Many synthetic and petroleum based ingredients require DEA to give them a favorable consistency and proper PH value.

1,4-Dioxane – This is an extremely carcinogenic chemical. In addition it is toxic to the entire non reproductive organ system in the body. It is a main component of Agent Orange, which was used extensively during the Vietnam War and thought to be the main culprit causing a host of cancers in US Military Vietnam Veterans. In woman it mimics estrogen in a bad way and therefore linked to causing Breast Cancer. Canada bans its use in any form in skin care products. In the United States it is so commonly used in producing petroleum based chemicals that the EWG (Environmental Working Group) found that it showed up in 50% of all skin care products they tested. It has also been found in over 65% of baby care cleansers and 60% of facial/body cleansers for women.

Polycyclic Aromatic Hydrocarbons (PAH) – PAH's are both carcinogenic and toxic. Like 1,4-Dioxane, PAH's are banned in Canada but not in the USA. It is an Endocrine System disruptor and organ system toxin. It is persistent and bioaccumulative. Once it is in your system it doesn't go away. It exists in thousands of skin care products with petroleum based chemicals including mineral oil and petrolatum.

Ethylene Oxide – This chemical is used for a process called Ethoxylation which is used to make certain chemicals, like Sodium Lauryl Sulfates in cleansing liquids to become more foaming and at the same time less abrasive. Ethylene Oxide by itself is extremely toxic to virtually all organs in the body. In addition it is usually the reason that 1,4-Dioxane (See Above) forms during the manufacturing of a multitude of skin care ingredients including PEG Stearates, Polysorbate-20, Dimethicone, Ceteareth-20, Caster Oil, etc. which in turn is used in tens of thousands of skin care products. Although it is used in the processing of thousands of chemicals that most people are not aware of, if the chemical has an "eth" in its name, stay away from it. That means it has gone through an Ethoxylation process.

Fragrance/Parfume – As noted in the previous chapter it is a catch all term that can contain upwards of 200 toxic/ carcinogenic chemicals including phthalates, parabens, and toluenes.

Arsenic – If your skin care product contains aluminum starch or cottonseed oil it could be contaminated with arsenic. Needless to say, arsenic is toxic and cancerous.

There are countless other hidden ingredients that exist in skin care formulations: way too many to list and would only complicate the issue if we did list them.

The point of this chapter is not an attempt to make you a knowledgeable chemist but to make you a knowledgeable consumer.

The ingredient list doesn't tell you everything that is in the bottle. But one thing it always tells you is if it contains synthetic chemicals. That being the case, you can be pretty sure it contains toxic hidden ingredients.

CHAPTER THIRTEEN
THE MORE YOU PAY – THE MORE THE TOXICITY

SYNTHETICS ARE SINFUL

As I reviewed various skin care products sold in this country I started noticing a consistency – not always true but mostly true. The higher cost products contained the highest levels of toxic chemicals. At first this seems completely paradoxical with what one would assume to be the complete opposite. Especially when one realizes that the most expensive skin care products are sold in top end spas, skin care centers, and doctors' offices. In fact, many of the expensive products are even sold under Doctor's names.

But then again, the more I investigated the more I realized this was not paradoxical, it was totally logical.

If somebody is willing to pay top dollar for a skin care product they expect top dollar results and they expect it to happen quickly.

How does someone make a skin care product give quick results? This was discussed to some degree in previous chapters.

No natural healthy unaltered Mother Nature ingredient is going to dissolve your wrinkles in 15 minutes. It may start to do it in 15 days, but not 15 minutes. Alas, the impatient client paying upwards of $100 an ounce for XYZ Elite Brand is not going to wait 15 days.

By filling the jar with higher concentrations of synthetic chemicals that will alter the skin cells, dramatically plump up the epidermis to disappear wrinkles, bleach the skin to rid it of dark spots, plasticize the skin surface to give sheen and smoothness is just the answer. Why worry about the harmful side effects or the fact that all the improvements disappear in short shrift once the chemicals either wear off or are destroyed by anti-bodies building up in the client?

The product was advertised to give you instant results and instant results you got.

Just because some product is branded under some doctors' name it doesn't mean it's any better or safer or healthier than a non-doctor brand. First of all, many of the so called Doctors' brands are not formulated by the Doctor's name on the bottle or any other doctor. They are formulated by chemical companies that offer "so called" private labeling products. In other words, the supplying chemical company develops, produces and packages the product using a label with the Doctors' name on it. That same exact formula may be packaged for another doctor with his name on it and so on and so on. Same product. Same manufacturer. Different name. This is common and done throughout the country and the world.

Private labeling is also done for Spas, Skin Med centers, Specialty cosmetic stores, etc.

Here is one case that you don't always get better by paying more. Be aware. Be clear.

CHAPTER FOURTEEN
PROCESSING – THE HEAT IS ON

SYNTHETICS ARE SINFUL

As stated in my Bio; Chemical Processing is my specialty. I spent over 30 years developing, installing and perfecting the most advanced processing equipment in the world for companies around the world. It was during that period that I saw what many companies did, including skin care manufacturers, that destroyed their product, introduced containments, and rendered much of the end product ineffective.

As much as I worry about using synthetic chemicals in any product, I get doubly worried about the processing method. I believe that it is in the processing, which is required by all synthetic chemicals that causes most of the harm to the human body. Whether it is beauty care products put on the outside of the body or processed food put inside the body, it all starts with processing methods.

This is where those toxic processing chemicals are added into the product and due to chemical reactions from that process, new and even more toxic chemicals are formed as a byproduct. All sitting in that jar that you take home from your store or spa.

Most skin care companies – large or small: local or foreign – use the same type of manufacturing processes. There are always exceptions, but the majority, almost 90% majority do the same or worse bad things. Even of more concern is the fact that many of those brand name products you bring home are not even made by the company listed on the jar.

When making beauty creams, the average formulation consists of mainly water up to 65%, followed by synthetic chemicals up to 35% and the remainder being natural Mother Nature ingredients.

Depending on what the chemical consistency is will determine which chemicals are mixed first and which are added last.

However, regardless of that, the basic processing involves mixing the water with emulsifying agents so that the water will then combine with the oils in the formula. In many cases the emulsification process requires heating the solution up in order to create a chemical reaction to occur. There are some emulsification processes that do not require heating.

In virtually all cases the product mixture will be subjected to heat for other reasons. The product is going to end up being a cream which means it is a semi solid. In order to homogenize and ensure thorough mixing takes place it is easier to bring the temperature up during processing so that all the ingredients become liquid.

Liquids are easier to mix and also easier to move through pipes to go from one mixing vat to another as chemicals are being added. It also is easier to fill up jars with a liquid than it is to fill it up when the product is in a semi solid cream state. The standard temperature to liquefy is around 165 degrees F.

This is where the problems begin. If there are any natural ingredients or organic botanical ingredients in the formula, they are damaged at this point.

It is much more convenient to ship product from regional warehouses than it is to ship it from one location which may be hundreds, if not thousands of miles away from the store it is going to. Sometimes companies opt to have their product made by regional formulator plants that are third party operators making products for several companies. Some formulators have better processing controls than the major brands they are manufacturing for, some have worse. As a customer you will never know.

At about 118 degrees, virtually all natural/organic oils get destroyed. At this temperature the vitamins, nutrients, bioflavonoids and enzymes either get cooked out or genetically altered so they are no longer able to do what they were intended to do. At 165 degrees the damage is much worse.

The USDA Organic guidelines only refer to what is being put into solution, it makes no statements about heat processing or other procedures. Even a totally organic product will be totally ineffective once heated above 118 degrees.

Even when heat is not required for proper mixing and homogenization, companies will normally heat for the filling stations. Companies want to make their packaging be attractive. Good looks sells better than ugly looks. When creams are going into fancy tubes or sculptured bottles with narrow openings, the automatic filling equipment almost requires a liquid for fast filling. Once it's in the jar the liquid cools down and solidifies. Now you have two problems.

The first problem is what we mentioned above, any good ingredients have been cooked out to become bad ingredients, devoid of virtually all its incumbent nutritional value. The unhealthy synthetic chemicals will still perform and invoke nasty side effects, but the healthy natural ingredients are left useless or worse, they can be carbonized to a harmful state.

The second problem is that most products, even the most expensive products are packaged in plastic tubes or jars. Plastics contains lots of toxins. Don't be fooled by companies that claim their plastics are BPA (Bisphenol A) free. Much of the concern surrounding plastic products these days is centered around bisphenol-A (BPA), a plastics chemical that numerous studies have found disrupts proper hormonal function, is linked to cancer and interferes with proper sexual development, among numerous other health issues.

But many plastics also contain phthalates, a known family of toxins which are more dangerous than BPA. In addition, plastics can contain xenoestrogens (hormonal disrupters), lead and antimony BPA free does not mean the plastic is toxin free.

When you pour 165 degree F liquid into a plastic jar you greatly increase the amount of toxins that leach out of the plastic right into that skin care cream you just bought and are about to infect and infuse into your body.

At my company we never heat our ingredients and we use virtually no plastic packaging. Since our cold fusion processing is proprietary, it is exclusive to us. But at the least, when you are buying beauty products, stay away from plastic containers and products that contain water and synthetic chemicals whenever you can.

CHAPTER FIFTEEN
MOTHER NATURE
NURTURES THE SKIN

SYNTHETICS ARE SINFUL

We have spent a lot of time explaining what is dangerous and does not work. Let's now talk about what does work and is healthy for the skin as well as the body and the mind.

Throughout this book I have told you about the dangers and side effects of synthetic chemicals. If you eliminate synthetic chemicals and the water that requires using synthetic chemicals then you eliminate virtually all of the down side of beauty care products and focus on the upside, the healthy side, the beneficial side, the healing side.

I do understand that some people are allergic to some of Mother Nature's plants and foods. That is quite minor compared to the fact virtually all people are allergic to synthetic chemicals. Most people know which foods/plants/oils that they are allergic to and can avoid using products that contain them since the names of those items are clearly identifiable in the ingredient list. That's not true with synthetic ingredients. Most people don't know what those chemicals are or what they contain.

Unprocessed Mother Nature's ingredients are easily identifiable when the producer states that the ingredients are "cold pressed" oils and/or Organic in nature. You want to buy a product that consist of only or at least mainly these ingredients. You don't want products with water or unrecognizable ingredient names or has added in vitamins which are usually always synthetic.

We talked about synthetic vitamins in previous chapters. Man can make ascorbic acid which has the same chemical formulation as Vitamin C. What Man cannot do is infuse synthetic ascorbic acid with nutrients, bioflavonoids or enzymes. The nutrients and bioflavonoids is what enhances Vitamin C and gives it potency. Enzymes are like the engines that drive the vitamins into the cells. Without enzymes the vitamin just passes through the body and does virtually nothing.

The human body does not produce Vitamin C, but Mother Nature does produce it with all the necessary constituents to make it work on the human body via many foods and plants, as well as in some animals.

This is true of all vitamins. When sourced from Mother Nature they work, when sourced from synthetic chemicals, they will not work and actually can become harmful.

When you buy a skin care product, make sure all of the vitamins are shown as being derived from plants or whole foods.

Make sure you read the ingredient list. The higher the percentage of organic botanical (plant) oils, the better the product. You want to see Mother Nature plants at the top of the list, or preferably the only things on the list period.

Your body will receive these ingredients the same way a sports car engine receives high octane cleansed gasoline. It will fire up the human engine and accelerate it to perform like never before.

I have made sure that whenever I formulate any of my skin care products, all of the ingredients are produced by Mother Nature. She is my only ingredient supplier.

It is very important that these ingredients are not heated above 118 degrees F and never processed with synthetic chemicals. Clean, Green and Lean are the rules for healthy effective Mother Nature formulations.

For your information I have listed below some of the more beneficial botanical oils that are used in healthy skin care products. The list is far from complete but at least serves as a starting point. Needless to say all oils are better for you when they are Organic and Pure.

Aloe Vera Extract - One of the most commonly known benefits of vitamin rich Aloe Vera Gel is its ability to soothe sunburned skin. Regular Aloe Vera gel is 99% water which is why you want to use the extract which is a concentrated form eliminating most of the water. Studies suggest that the polysaccharides in Aloe Vera might protect against non-melanoma type skin cancers by targeting pathways activated by ultra violet radiation. Ultra violet radiation suppresses the body's natural immune responses and causes premature aging. It also aids in fighting psoriasis. Aloe Vera absorbs into the skin almost four times faster than water – making it an excellent moisturizer and emollient. Its antimicrobial properties kill bacteria and its anti-inflammatory abilities make it a great solution for those with oily skin who may also suffer with acne. The rapid stretching in skin causes small tears (commonly called "stretch marks") that Aloe Vera can help heal and prevent. Aloe Vera contains antioxidant vitamins A, C and E as well as vitamin B12 and folic acid along with eight enzymes several minerals such as calcium, copper, selenium, chromium, manganese, magnesium, potassium, sodium and zinc.

Apricot Kernel Seed Oil – This oil is a light and gentle oil used in creams, lotions and other beauty products to balance, nourish and lubricate your skin. It is rich in gamma linoleic acid, or GLA, which comes from essential fatty acid omega-6. The GLA content in apricot kernel oil helps skin to maintain moisture balance. GLA also plays a role in firming and toning your skin. Additionally, organic apricot kernel oil contains vitamin A and E, which soothe the skin and slow signs of aging. The nourishing properties of apricot kernel seed oil have an anti-inflammatory effect and may soothe minor skin conditions such as eczema.

Avocado Oil: Due to its high vitamin and nutritional content, avocado oil assists in collagen production which gives firmness and wrinkle resistance to the skin. It has a natural capability of retaining water which gives a softness and moisturizing effect to the skin. It contains Vitamin A in the healthiest and most anti-ageing/ anti-oxidant natural form, as Beta Carotene. Additionally, it contains nutritional potassium. The sterolins in Avacado Oil lessen blemishes while relieving UV ray damaged skin. These sterolins also enhance immune function through absorbing fat and lowering incidence of skin damage. Avocado oil has a high content of Vitamin E that helps to eliminate free radicals and decelerate the signs of ageing.

Camelina Oil *(Camelina Sativa):* - Camelina is also known as wild flax. It has been domesticated and extensively used in Europe for several thousand years. Camelina Oil contains omega-3 fatty acids, as well as a unique antioxidant complex including tocopherols (vitamin E), carotenoids (Vitamin A), and phosphatides (Lecithin). Phosphatides are great hydrating elements for the skin.

Camellia Oil - It is an excellent emollient for dry skin. It not only moisturizes, but because it is readily absorbed it prevents and smooths out wrinkles. It has been known to help with acne. The Biosafety Research Center for Foods in Japan have found that Camellia oil inhibits melanoma (skin cancers). Camellia plants grow in East Asia and China. It contains Vitamins A, B, C, E and Polyphenol which are all natural anti-oxidants. It aids in diminishing or eliminating fine lines, pitted acne scarring and the appearance of large pores.

Coconut Oil – This oil quickly melts and penetrates into the skin to moisturize, nourish and soften the skin. Along with its Oleic Acids which energizes skin cell generation it also contains high amounts of Vitamin E which is a super anti-oxidizing agent. Coconut Oil is a natural SPF oil which when combined with Shea Butter increases its protection factor against sun damage and wrinkling.

Grapeseed Oil - It is light and therefore is easily absorbed into the skin. Rather than using harmful alcohols, Grapeseed Oil is a great penetrant and serves to carry other ingredients in the lotion safely and without alteration into the skin. It is a good moisturizer. It also has an astringent property to aid in the tightening and toning of the skin. It is especially effective around the eyes. This oil is rich in vitamin C and E, and Beta Carotene which the body converts into a natural and safe form of vitamin A. Grapeseed oil also contains some essential fatty acids. It has been used in treating Acne and other skin ailments.

Hemp Seed Oil - It is considered to be one of the most nutritional oils available. It contains all three essential fatty acids in the right proportions for the human body (Omega 3, Omega 6 and Omega 9) to promote a healthy luster to the skin, hair and eyes. It contains all twenty known amino acids, including the nine essential amino acids that aid in firming up skin and fighting wrinkles. It is a natural anti-oxidant. It also contains Vitamins A, B1, B2, B3, B6, C, D & E. It has been used to assist in skin conditions such as Eczema, Psoriasis, and Acne as well as many other medical conditions.

Jojoba Oil - It is excellent for supplementing the treating and resolving of acne and blemishes. It has a rich content of vitamin E that helps in preventing wrinkles on the skin. It acts as a natural antioxidant too. It is effective in bringing down skin inflammations and is capable of killing some skin bacteria. Jojoba oil provides the required moisture to the skin without blocking the skin pores. It is quickly absorbed into the skin giving it a hydrating effect and an improvement of the blood flow which adds to skin glow. It has a striking similarity with human sebum, the oily substance responsible for giving a smooth effect to our skin and hair. Thus it works well on both dry and oily skin since it acts as sebum balancer. Because it is hypoallergenic it can be used even on skin that has eruptions.

Kukui Nut Oil - The Kukui Tree is the official state tree of Hawaii providing a quick absorbing oil with high penetrability into even the deepest layers of the skin. It moisturizes and offers a protective shield from the atmospheric elements of sun and wind. It aids in fighting Eczema, Psoriasis and Acne. It contains essential fatty acids and natural anti-oxidants in the form of Vitamin A, C, and E.

Lavender Essential Oil - Its skin benefits include that of being antiseptic and anti-fungal which helps to reduce scarring and speeds healing of acne, wrinkles, psoriasis, and inflammation. When bacteria are kept in check the skin stays healthier and more vibrant. Lavender essential oil is also an anti-inflammatory and circulatory stimulant. Stimulating circulation increases blood flow and brings more nutrients to keep the skin cells healthier. By being anti-inflammatory it helps to reduce skin blotchiness. The Lavender scent is also aromatheraputic which can help reduce stress.

Lemon Essential Oil – This oil has been historically recognized as a cleanser. It is reputed as being antiseptic, and as having refreshing and cooling properties. The aromatheraputic properties of Lemon Essential Oil is to enhance the ability to concentrate. Lemon Oil is a natural skin toning agent.

Meadowfoam Oil - This oil contains over 98% of long chain fatty acids (Brassic, Erucic, and Gadoleic) that is extremely stable and prevents the skin from seeing moisture loss. It protects against Ultra-violet rays and gives sunscreen protection. Meadowfoam acts as a natural preservative without any toxic formaldehydes that are used in synthetic preservatives. It soaks into the skin easily and moisturizes from within.

Olive Oil – It contains three major antioxidants: vitamin E, polyphenols, and phytosterols. Antioxidants fight free radicals which damage skin cells and are a major cause of aging skin. Vitamin E not only is an antioxidant it also helps to restore skin smoothness as well as protecting against ultraviolet light damage. Olive Oil contains Hydroxytyrosol which is an extremely rare compound that greatly enhances its ability to stop free radical damage to the skin. Olive Oil never clogs the pores instead it quickly penetrates the skin serving as a great carrier agent for other ingredients and cleans the pores as it passes through them.

Orange Essential Oil – This essential oil has shown to promote the production of collagen as well as increase the blood flow to the skin adding natural luster. It is helpful at soothing dry, irritated skin as well as acne-prone skin. It is excellent for rubbing on calluses on the feet. In Aromatherapy it used to sooth the mind and helps to relieve stress.

Pumpkin Seed Oil – Pumpkin Seed Oil is known to provide moisturizing properties to dry and damaged skin. This is because of its high levels of Omega 3, 6 and 9 fatty acids. Combining that with its content of Vitamin E antioxidant properties to fight free radicals and zinc, Pumpkin seed oil helps the skin to retain moisture, maintain a youthful skin tone and help healing of bad cells. There is a plethora of additional minerals and vitamins to aid in its anti-aging effects.

Rosehip Seed Oil - Besides having a mix of essential fatty acids, Rosehip also contains Vitamin A in its natural form as Tretinoin, and Vitamin C. This helps to delay effects of skin aging and assists in cell regeneration and promoting collagen and elastin levels to increase. Rosehip Oil has been independently tested with excellent results. One test in 1983 in Santiago Chile by the University of Santiago was conducted on 180 individuals with extensive facial scarring, acne scarring, deep wrinkles, sun damage, and deep wrinkles. The results proved the effectiveness of Rosehip Seed Oil to aid in resolving those conditions. In 1988, Dr. Bertha Pareja and Dr. Kehl, both pharmacologists did a test on 20 women, aged 20 to 35. Within 3 weeks of using Rosehip Oil significant improvements on brown spots, wrinkles, and eye lids affected by UV damage were noted. At the end of four months, virtually all the brown spots and surface wrinkles had disappeared.

Sacha Inchi Oil: This oil is harvested from the Sacha Inchi Nut which is indigenous to the Peruvian Rain Forest. Many health experts refer to Sacha Inchi as a superfood for both the body and the skin. The reason being that Sacha Inchi has the highest content of Omega 3, 6 and 9 than any other source on earth – animal, mineral or vegetable. Sacha Inchi Oil contains 15 times the amount of Omega 3 of an equivalent amount of Salmon. Your skin and body requires all three of these Omega's which is why they are called the Essential Fatty Acids (EFA's). Sachi Inchi Oil is 48% Omega 3, 36% Omega 6 and 8% Omega 9. Your body can produce its own Omega 9 but it cannot synthesize or produce Omega 3 and/or Omega 6. Yet, Omega 3 is the most critical and beneficial EFA for your skin. EFA's are needed to manufacture and repair cell membranes. To maximize and activate the benefits of Omega 3 your body needs an additional 50% to 75% Omega 6. Sacha Inchi provides the perfect ratio of both Omega's. This enables the cells to reach optimum nutrition and expel harmful byproducts at the same time. Strong membranes also allow the cells to maintain water with minimal evaporation which gives the skin a full and wholesome look. In addition, research on Omega 3 has found that it protects against cancer, viral infections and builds up the immune system for healthy looking skin. Sachi Inchi is also rich in iodine, vitamin A and vitamin E which makes it a strong anti-oxidant and wrinkle fighter.

Shea Butter – This butter is derived from the Karite or Shea Tree grown in West Africa. It has been claimed to be the richest of all butters. Not all Shea Butters are the same. Although more expensive and rarer, it is best to use hand crafted shea butter which is never heated or gas pressurized to remove it from the shell. It is naturally rich in Vitamins A, E, and F, as well as a number of other vitamins and minerals. Vitamins A and E help to soothe, hydrate, and balance the skin. They also stimulate the skin to generate more collagen which assists with reducing wrinkles and other signs of ageing. Vitamin F contains essential fatty acids, and helps protect and revitalize damaged skin and hair. Vitamin F also helps to produce elastin which gives the skin its elasticity and youthful appearance. Shea Butter is an intense moisturizer for dry skin, and is a wonderful product for revitalizing dull or dry skin on the body or scalp. It promotes skin renewal, increases the circulation, and accelerates wound healing. It also offers a natural SPF (between5 and 10) against damaging sun UV rays. It is excellent for dry skin, stretch marks, damaged skin and sunburn.

Sunflower Oil - Lots of Oleic (Omega 3) fatty acids combined high amounts of Vitamin A, D, and E. The Vitamin A is in the healthy cartonoid form which is a great anti-wrinkle deterrent. The high amounts of Vitamin E fight free radical damage to skin cells It also contains lecithin which is essential for healthy skin cell function. It aids the intake of healthy nutrients into the cells and the discharge of unhealthy substances. It is quickly absorbed into the skin and is an excellent carrier and penetrates to deeper layers. It is an anti-oxidant. The phospholipids in lecithin naturally attract water from the air which aids in hydrating the skin. Folic acid is present in Sunflower Oil which aids the body to manufacture new cells.

CHAPTER SIXTEEN
CAN A SUNSCREEN
PROMOTE MELANOMA

Before we talk about the sunscreens themselves, let's talk about what we are trying to screen against.

The Sun puts out three major types of ultra violet light: UVA, UVB and UVC. We don't have to address UVC since the ionosphere stops all UVC before it reaches the Earth. UV stands for Ultra Violet and although it is considered a form of light, it consists of waves that are so short it is not visible to the human eye. It's all around us, but we can't see it.

UVA – This is the most abundant form of UV rays and represents approximately 95% of all the UV rays reaching the earth. Although less potent than UVB it is more penetrating. UVA can easily pass through glass including car windshields. It has both a short wave and a long wave component for deep penetration into the skin. Think of UV(A) for aging. It is the major cause of wrinkling and damage below the epidermis. It is the UVA that damages cells below the skin surface and can destroy your collagen. UVA rays can damage your immune system and thereby reduce your ability to prevent melanoma from occurring.

UVB – The UVB rays are the most potent to reach the earth. They are not as penetrating as UVA (i.e. they cannot pass through glass) but they are more powerful. Think of UV(B) for burning. It is the major cause of sunburn, tanning and skin cancer. It is also the major contributor to absorption and conversion of Vitamin D in the body.

Herein is the paradox, UV rays can cause skin cancer, but they are the major producer of Vitamin D for the body which is what we need to fight cancer. Our body is not able to produce Vitamin D unless we are exposed to UV rays. Yes, we can get some Vitamin D by eating dark berries and some other foods, but we cannot eat enough of anything to produce the amount of Vitamin D we need to protect our body. Only the sun's UV rays can do that.

This is one of the problems with sunscreens, they block the very rays we need to produce Vitamin D so we can protect ourselves from those same rays. A little confusing, yes, but let's move on and maybe we can unconfused it.

The previous paragraph gives a hint of explanation as to the fact that as use of sunscreens increase like they have over the last 50 years; the occurrence of skin cancer has also increased at an alarming rate. Skin cancer is one of the fastest growing cancers in the USA.

However, there is a more devious reason for the increase of skin cancer than just the fact we are reducing our Vitamin D production, it is the sunscreen itself that induces cancer.

Unfortunately, the same lack of regulation for beauty products has been transferred to sunscreens. Actually it is worse for sunscreens.

Let's correct the myths, misleading information and outright lies told to the public.

Most people think if they buy a sunscreen with an SPF (Sun Protection Factor) of 60, it will give them double the protection of a sunscreen with an SPF of 30 and they can stay out in the sun twice as long. Well, that is totally untrue.

The SPF is not really a measure of how much time you can spend in the sun, it is a measure of what percentage of the UVB rays it prevents from reaching your skin. Please note, SPF says nothing about the protection against UVA rays. It only is a measure of UVB protection regardless of what the company puts on their brochure.

I have seen companies talk about their SPF cream giving you UVA/UVB protection. Sometimes they talk about their product giving you a UVA/UVB blended or "broad spectrum" protection. In the USA as of the year 2016, that is outright misleading at best, and a total lie in reality. All SPF ratings are based on UVB blockage only. If they produce a cream that gives SPF (30) protection for UVB rays and SPF (1) protection for UVA rays, they can call it SPF (30) UVA/UVB broad spectrum protection. The UVA rays will pass right through the sunscreen and age you and attack you the same as if you had nothing on at all. What you want to look for on the literature, or call up and ask of the manufacturer is exactly what is the SPF for the UVA rays. If they won't or can't tell you the answer, then move on to another brand that will give you a breakdown of their SPF protection for each of the UV rays.

The USA is basically the only major country that still allows mislabeling of SPF protection.

An SPF 30 will stop 97% of the UVB rays from reaching your skin. SPF 50 blocks 98% and SPF 100 blocks 99%. That is only true if you apply enough of the sunscreen to your body.

When sunscreens are tested for SPF designation, the standard rule is to use 2.0 mg of product per cm^2 of surface area. In simple terms that means on the average body adorned in a swimming suit you would have to use at least one full ounce per application. It should also be understood that if the sunscreen is synthetically chemically based, those chemicals will break down under the sun's rays within 45 minutes and you must recoat your body with an additional ounce of cream for every 45 minutes that you are out in the sun. If you try to spread out the cream so you don't use as much up and save money, you will not be saving anything else, especially your skin.

Using ½ the proper amount of cream does not provide you ½ the protection, it provides you only ¼ the protection. Applying 1/3 the proper amount affords you 1/9 the protection. Your SPF protection goes from 30 to 3. If you don't reapply every 45 minutes, you will have zero protection. Even worse, the chemicals that were applied previously actually breakdown to a harmful state due to UV overload and can induce cancerous activity.

Using sunscreen all the time you are outside can promote cancer, including melanoma. You need to expose yourself to the sun for at least a short period on a regular basis. Recent studies have indicated that Vitamin D prevents up to 77% of all cancers including breast cancer, colon cancer, cervical cancer, lung cancer and brain tumors. People of African origin need to stay out in the sun even longer. The darker your skin, the longer you need to expose yourself to the sun, as much as 20 times more, in order to produce enough vitamin D.

If it hurts when you press your fingertips firmly on your Sternum (breast bone in the center of your rib cage) then you may be suffering from chronic vitamin D deficiency right now.

All through this book I have been stating that "SYNTHETICS ARE SINFUL". When it comes to sunscreens it is even worse. In the USA there are only 16 chemicals that are FDA approved for use in sunscreens. The one place where the FDA gets involved in sunscreens is approving chemicals that can be used. The one place where the FDA is slower than a turtle overdosing on sleeping tablets is approving chemicals for use in sunscreens. We are years behind Europe and Australia in developing and/or approving new, safer and more effective chemicals for sunscreen application. Europe has approved 27 chemicals to our 16. Europe has chemicals much more capable to protect you from both UVA and UVB rays then here.

Out of those 16 chemicals approved in the USA, only 6 are currently being used. Oxybenzone, avobenzone, octinoxate, octisalate, homosalate and octocrylene.

OXYBENZONE

The real problem is the fact that over 80% of the sunscreens sold in the USA use Oxybenzone as the main sunscreen protection ingredient. Oxybenzone has been banned since 1997 in Europe, Canada and Australia. This chemical has been found to be an endocrine disrupter, organ toxin and cell attacker. It is persistent which means it does not leave the body and the more you use the more you accumulate (bioaccumulative). It is a penetrant and therefore carries toxins deep into the body. It has a short life when exposed to UV rays and becomes virtually ineffective in blocking any UV rays within 45 to 60 minutes.

The other chemicals are not good for you either. They may not be as bad as Oxybenzone, but they certainly aren't good.

None of them give you a wide range of both UVA and UVB protection. Protect you they not.

Absorbing many of these chemicals through your skin is bad enough, but too many people want the convenience of a spray on sunscreen. This is the worst of the worst. It's bad enough letting these chemicals penetrate through your skin. When you use a spray you also inhale it directly into the body making it even more disruptive.

My strong advice and recommendation is not buying any sunscreen that uses chemicals as the sunscreen protectorate. Never use a spray on sunscreen.

Another product to avoid is a moisturizing cream that is combined with chemical sun blockers to achieve an SPF rating. Putting those two items in the same bottle means a lot of extra processing is being done to make the moisturizer and the sunscreen in a homogenized solution. Usually this takes away from the effectiveness of both and increases the toxicity of each.

If you want moisturizing and sunscreen protection, then put on your moisturizer first, let it sink in and then put your sunscreen cream on top of it.

You should try to stay out of the sun between 11 AM and 4 PM during the summer months. I know that won't work on a beach day, but you should consider using protective clothing and/or umbrellas when you are on the beach. Get a little sun on your body to get some Vitamin D absorption. When it comes time to put on a sunscreen I highly recommend you use only one type. No chemicals, just pure natural minerals.

ZINC OXIDE

Zinc Oxide is a natural mineral compound that offers the safest and widest range of UVA and UVB protection in the marketplace anywhere in the world. You still have to apply the same amount as required for chemicals, approximately one ounce at a time. However, zinc oxide does not have to be replaced as often and in any case, is not toxic to your body. Make sure you only buy zinc oxide products that state they are using non-nano (larger) sized particles. If the jar does not say non-nano then assume it is nano and stay away from it.

Zinc Oxide is a white compound. When properly formulated it will become transparent on the skin after a few minutes after application. The simple and less expensive way to make zinc oxide transparent is to process it down to very small particles in the nano (microscopic) size range. When this is done you shorten the protection range along with allowing these very small particles to dig deep down into your skin and accumulate there.

Sometimes sunscreens are formulated with both Zinc Oxide and chemical sun blockers. Do not use these. You do not want any sun block chemicals on your skin.

As far as SPF levels, I would recommend that you stay below SPF 50. Anything higher is not giving any additional protection of consequence and may contain more chemicals then you want.

Remember that sunburn occurs easier on skin with nutritional deficiencies that leave the skin vulnerable to DNA mutations from radiation. You can offer a lot of protection to your skin from what you eat as well as what you put on it. Eating lots of berries which contain anti-oxidant nutrition along with plant based vitamins and nutrients will maximize your sun protection and minimize damage.

For an informative video on the understanding of sunscreens and UV rays, go to YouTube and type in

Dr. Edward Gorham Skin Cancer/Sunscreen – The Dilemma.

This will bring you to a lecture that Dr. Gorham gave at University of California, San Diego Campus.

CHAPTER SEVENTEEN
LIPS, HAIR, NAILS AND SCENT

The main thrust of this book has been to focus on skin care products. That is my strongest area of expertise. I am not an expert by any means on products used for the lips, hair, nails or the perfumes used for scentifying oneself.

However, in my research and interfacing with individuals about skin care products I have come across some information about those products that I would like to pass on to you. It seems the lies, myths and misdirection is not just used on skin care products, it expands in other areas of the beauty industry as well.

Lipstick – The Kiss of Death

By carefully classifying what goes on your lips, stays on your lips, the cosmetic industry has been able to avoid, with the blessing of the FDA, any regulations that would pertain to an item that is ingested like a food. Evidently the FDA has determined that no woman who puts on lipstick has ever put their tongue on the various creams and paints used to protect and color those lips. They must also believe that when eating food every woman makes sure the food never touches their lips. Hey, what about the man in her life? They must assume that they never touch lips when kissing? Lipstick is not just a woman problem, it is a woman and lover problem.

According to a study released by the consumer activist group Campaign for Safe Cosmetics, more than 60% of 33 brand name lipsticks contain lead, but not a single label lists it as an ingredient. In fact, one major brand has 60 times more lead in it than what is allowed by law to be in paint for the wall. The FDA doesn't want you to lick lead off of your wall because it may be life threatening but it is OK to lick 60 times more lead off of your own lips. Quite insane.

Lead has been directly linked to Alzheimer's disease. More than 2/3 of people with Alzheimer's are women. Maybe a coincidence, but I would guess that all that lead in lipstick is not helping the situation.

Lip balms are just as bad, maybe worse. Some lip balms, some very popular lip balms advertised on TV with a major movie star contains polyethylene which is a known immune system toxin along with BHT which is a formaldehyde releaser. The longer you keep on the balm the more you add the toxin formaldehyde to your body. It is interesting that Balm is one half of the word Embalm.

A majority of lip balms use mineral oil and petrolatum as a major ingredient. As we mentioned previously, mineral oil contains the hidden ingredient 1,4-Dioxane which is toxic and carcinogenic.

Hair Dyes Are to Die For

It isn't like it hasn't been known for years that hair dyes are toxic. Back in 1987 Cornel University put together a Health Hazard Manual for Cosmetologists and Hairdressers because their research found that hairdressers have a much higher incidence of cancer and reproductive issues then the general population because of the chemicals in hair dyes and shampoos. Cornel found an additional 20% of hairdressers had to leave the profession due to health problems such as allergies and dermatitis. The same toxins that were in hair products back then are still in them today.

The hair shampoos contain SLS or sodium lauryl sulfates. SLS is derived from laural alcohol which is processed using ethoxylation. We talked about the ethoxylation process in Chapter 12 when discussing hidden ingredients. This process creates a byproduct of 1,4-dioxane which is toxic and carcinogenic. SLS and the contaminant 1,4-dioxane is in over 80% of shampoos, cleansers and baby soaps.

About 90% of hair dyes contain PPD (para-phenyllenediamine), a toxic substance which is highly carcinogenic and directly linked to lymph node cancer as well as breast cancer, leukemia and multiple myeloma. There are other toxins (APE's) which are hormonal disrupters.

The Harvard School of Public Health's epidemiology department discovered that women who use hair coloring more than five times annually are twice as likely to develop ovarian cancer. The International Cancer Journal found that women who use permanent hair coloring are twice as likely to get bladder cancer. The Cancer Prevention Coalition lists hair dyes as one of the most harmful consumer products.

I don't imagine women are going to stop coloring their hair, but I hope they will look for alternative hair dyes that don't contain PPD or APE chemicals.

Nail Polish – Nailing The Truth

This an easy one. Every nail salon you walk into you will see that all the manicurists wear masks. Could it be they know something we don't? A major problem with nail polish is that in order to keep it flexible after it hardens requires the use of a plasticizer. The two most populat plasticizers are phthalates and/or TPHP (triphenyl phosphate). Duke University joined forces with the Environmental Working Group (EWG) in 2015 and found that all women they tested contained and retained those chemicals in their bodies when tested for it 15 hours after they finished doing their nails.

Both phthalates and TPHP are endocrine/hormonal disruptors. The **endocrine system** is the collection of glands that produce hormones that regulate metabolism, growth and development, tissue function, sexual function, reproduction, sleep, and mood, among other things. Disrupting this system disrupts the entire body. The younger you are starting to disrupt the system; the more damage you receive.

Fragrances – The Sweet Poison

The term fragrance is the catch all for the highest concentration of toxins in any skin care product. Over 800 toxic compounds are used in the manufacturing of perfumes and upwards of 100 of those compounds can exist in any one product. With perfumes, the manufacturer wants it to last as long as possible so therefore they use penetrants to drop it deep into the skin, they use plasticizers to open up the pores, they use VOC's (Volatile Organic Compounds) to release the scent and phthalates to make the fragrance last as long as possible. These toxins enter the skin and the nose to fully encompass the body and penetrate those toxins through every avenue possible.

Let it suffice to say, use perfumes sparingly and only for special occasions. Frequent use will create more toxic infusion than you want or need.

CHAPTER EIGHTEEN
THE HEALTHY POSITIVE CONCLUSION

We certainly have reviewed a lot of the problems with skin care products, but hopefully those explanations have served to make you more aware and therefore able to make healthier decisions with better results in your search to keep your skin the best it can be.

In Chapter One I said that healthy skin is always more important than younger looking skin. In reality, healthy skin is the only way to achieve the youngest looking skin.

Please note that the first four letters of healthy spells "heal". Too many of the cosmetics we put on our face do not "heal" but instead, "disrupts". Disruption eventually leads to "damage" and then "destruction".

You only have one body. It's going to be with you your entire life. Treat it with the care it deserves so it can give you the life you deserve.

No matter how much makeup you put on: no matter how much skin creams you apply: no matter how many injections you do to your skin, if your skin is not healthy it won't look well. I truly believe that surface beauty is driven by the real beauty from underneath.

Although we have not discussed the foods we put in our body it is an intricate part of keeping our outer body healthy.

Life is about decisions. The decisions we make today will always determine what tomorrow will bring.

When it comes to deciding what to put on your skin, remember you are also deciding what is going into your skin, your body and your organs.

Do not let some uncaring third party, like some skin care product providers driven by profit instead of promise, make those decisions for you. Arm yourself with knowledge, because knowledge is power.

This book only touches the surface of what you can learn and understand about the Beauty Industry and what they are putting into their products.

The web provides an additional wealth of knowledge. Just make sure you go to credible, unbiased, honest providers of that knowledge. I have mentioned some of them in the chapters above. I certainly feel that the Environmental Working Group (ewg.org) is a fantastic and honest source for that knowledge.

I started formulating skin care products to protect my family, I started Replenish Plus to serve the public, I wrote this book to inform you.

I wish you a healthy and happy future: filled with an absence of toxic chemicals and a deluge of nutritional substances.

STAY HEALTHY - STAY YOUNG

REFERENCES

This is the part of the book where most Authors want to list as many sources as possible with as many recognizable names and institutes in order to provide credibility to their own writings. I have decided to take a different direction because it would be impossible for me to list all the sources who have given me the resources and knowledge to write this book. My references are the thousands of people I have met in the industry over a thirty-year period traveling across the world. Information came to me not just from the Scientists and Engineers working in Labs, but also from formulators, processing people and maintenance personnel working in the plants actually making and developing products. It did not just come from the hundreds of theoretical papers and University studies that I read which sometimes came to conclusions not justified by the reality, but it also came from the writings and records and procedures of companies and people actually making product and testing the results that I had access to during my career as a chemical processing equipment developer. This book is the result of thousands of notes, millions of words and countless interactions with the Corporate Officers, Scientists, Engineers, Office Workers and Maintenance People that I had the good fortune to meet while traveling to over 40 countries and working in thousands of plants around the world. These are my references; these are my sources and resources of factual information; these are the people to whom I thank for teaching me and allowing me to have the knowledge to put together this book.

Printed in the United States
By Bookmasters